Proud Flesh

Sex, God, and the Redemptive Power of Flat Foot Dancing

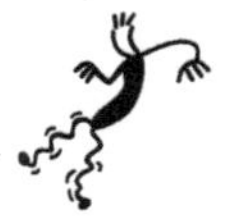

Ginger T. Manley

Ideas into Books®
WESTVIEW
Kingston Springs, Tennessee

Ideas into Books®
WESTVIEW
P.O. Box 605
Kingston Springs, TN 37082
www.ideasintobooks.net

ISBN: 978-1-62880-072-2 Perfect Bound
ISBN 978-1-62880-074-6 Smashwords
ISBN 978-1-62880-075-3 Amazon Kindle

First edition, April 2016

Photo credits: The back cover photograph is from the author's private collection.

Cover design by Eddie Patton of The Wanderer Company.

Printed in the United States of America on acid free paper.

Other books by Ginger Manley

Gotcha Covered: A Legacy of Service and Protection, 2009, Published by Westview, Inc. Available in soft cover through Internet retailers and in select book sellers.

Assisted Loving: The Journey through Sexuality and Aging, 2013, Published by Westview, Inc. Available through Internet retailers in soft cover and eBook versions.

Disarmed: An Exceptional Journey, 2015, *Ideas into Books*® WESTVIEW. Available through Internet retailers in soft cover and eBook versions.

Other publications and information are available at http://www.gingermanley.com.

Ginger Manley can be contacted at ginger@gingermanley.com.

Trixie blogs at www.proudfleshbook.com.

...And see how the flesh grows back across a wound, with a great vehemence,

more strong than the simple, untested surface before. There's a name for it on horses, when it comes back darker and raised: proud flesh

...Jane Hirshfield, "For What Binds Us"

PART ONE: Prologue

October 1992

Chicago

"Who'd have thought something left in an old Brownie camera for almost forty years could still be developed?" Frances Murphy said to the clerk in the film lab.

Handing her the change from her twenty-dollar bill, the young man smiled and nodded. "Yes, ma'am. We get these old rolls of film from time to time. As long as it's black and white and it's been stored inside a house instead of an attic or a garage, we can usually get good results."

Later, sitting in her small north side apartment with an untouched cup of tea cooling in its porcelain cup and saucer nearby, Frances propped up the photograph on the table next to her chair. Merging herself with the image of the man and his adoring daughter smiling at each other in front of the fireplace, she whispered, "I know it's not your way, Art, but I have to do this. If I don't clean up the past then I can't clear up my future."

She picked up the felt-tipped pen and spiral-bound notebook she had purchased after leaving the photo store. "For Carroll's Eyes Only" she wrote in bold letters on the cover, the uneven characters betraying her anxiety, then opening to the first lined notebook page she wrote,

Oct. 29, 1992

Dearest Carroll,

Happy 46th Birthday! How I wish I could say these words directly to you instead of putting them in my journal. You've not accepted anything I've mailed you for more than twenty-five years, so I had quit writing, even in this form, for a long time while I was feeling so low, but now I'm ready to start again.

The past four years have been hard for me. I guess it's because I was dreading the prospect of turning seventy, but I became quite depressed during this time. I'd always had trouble sleeping and needed to take prescriptions to help, but I denied to my doctors that anything was wrong with me. I began to drink more heavily, and finally I had to come to the realization I was an addict. Addict was so hard for me to say about myself. I felt so ashamed of getting to this point in my life and letting myself lose control in such a way.

But one day my friend Midge, Janie's mother, came over when I wasn't expecting her and she found I hadn't bathed or dressed for several days and could barely even say my name. She told me she was giving me an ultimatum—either I would agree to go to the Betty Ford Center or she would call my brother or my pastor and tell them what she'd found. I was desperate, so I went to Betty Ford and it was the best thing I've ever done for myself. I'd have given anything if you'd been there for family week, but you refused to take any of the calls made to you. Uncle Morton and Aunt Belle came out, and it was wonderful to start to clear up so much old baggage. I still hold hope that one day I'll see you in person again. If it's not to be, then maybe someday you'll read my journal.

You are my precious beloved child,

Love always,

Mother

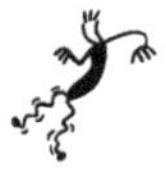

November 1992

Nashville airport

Carroll Murphy really needed to pee by the time her plane from Los Angeles landed in Nashville. In fact, finding a toilet was about the only thing on her mind as she deplaned and headed to the restroom. All her life she had been fussy about public toilets, and she particularly hated those tiny airplane johns.

As she eased into a squat, she congratulated herself once more for giving up wearing pantyhose, which were a terrible inconvenience in bathrooms. The squat was a remnant from her childhood training, which no manner of adult logic could change for Carroll. *Don't sit down on a toilet seat that's not at our house*, Carroll would hear in her mind, knowing it was the voice of Frances, her mother, implanted in her when she was a child.

You'd think I could make up my own mind about such things. After all, I am an adult now, Carroll would tell herself, to no avail. Even as a fiercely independent professional woman more than halfway through her forties, she still could not lower herself to sit on an unfamiliar toilet seat.

Oh well, she would sigh. *At least it keeps my thighs toned.*

With relief, she leaned to adjust her knee-highs before pulling up the tailored gabardine slacks she was wearing, and she smiled a little to hear the comforting gurgle of the automatic flush.

I can't believe this—Nashville plumbing is even ahead of Newark, now, Carroll thought, remembering her recent bathroom adventure in that airport where travelers had not flushed their own waste and the stench was becoming intolerable. *I don't think they even had flush toilets when I lived in this backwoods town twenty-nine years ago*, she thought, shaking her head a little.

She waited to wash her hands in line behind two women who were planted in front of the sinks. Peering over them, she watched as the younger one—probably the daughter—helped the older one, who was seated in a wheelchair, keep her hands under the automatic faucet long enough for the water to begin to flow.

Am I really seeing what I think I'm seeing? Unbelievable! Carroll thought, shaking her head.

A cap made of plastic six-pack drink holders crocheted together in bright orange and white yarn covered the thinning gray hair of the older woman, who Carroll guessed to be about Medicare age. The daughter wore a hat that was an exact copy of her mother's. Graying roots tipped with henna peeked out from under the brim of the hat and a face of cracked glass betrayed the daughter's attempt to conceal the fact that in about fifteen or so years she would also be receiving her *Welcome to Medicare* card from the government.

"Don't make no sense to me, why they got to have these newfangled automagic things. Seems like a body could at least turn it on and off herself," the older woman wheezed to the younger one, who by then was intently peering into the mirror, plucking at a pesky coarse hair from the rather large mole on her chin.

"Ruby Lee, I swear, these modern contraptions are enough to make a person 'bout croak on the spot," spoke the mother, still trying to get both soap and water on her ancient hands at the same time.

"Now don't git yoreself so worked up, Ma. Yore asthma will give yoreself fits if you're a-fussing," Ruby Lee instructed.

She leaned over and adjusted the oxygen tube entering her mother's nostrils, gently looping the plastic tubing back over her ears. Her mother shot Ruby Lee a scornful look and tugged the tube off her ears, letting it dangle on her neck before it found its way to the hospital-green canister of compressed air supported in its trolley on the floor. Satisfied they had both accomplished all they could in the restroom, Ruby Lee turned her mother's wheelchair and oxygen tank towards the exit sign and threaded their way out through the incoming throng of women.

Carroll finished washing her hands and then tweaked her hair slightly to confirm that her own roots were not showing. She leaned in to the mirror to repair her lipstick and smiled at her reflection, knowing she and Ruby Lee would never be mistaken for contemporaries. Exiting the restroom, she crossed the corridor to the TCBY kiosk and bought a small cone of sugar-free strawberry yogurt. With several minutes to kill before she had to re-board the plane, she also picked up the current *Time* magazine.

MANDATE FOR CHANGE screamed the cover in two-inch bold letters displayed under the jutting jaw of the newly elected president. *What Will Clinton Do?* ran the subtitle. Flipping through the pages, she smiled to note her presidential candidate had won with more western, more female, more single, more moderate, and more white votes than had past Democratic winners. *Guess my vote mattered*, she mused.

Carroll was just taking the last bite of her cone when she spotted the pair from the restroom waiting for the same Orlando-bound plane as she. Ruby Lee had finished devouring a cinnamon bun and a few flakes of its sugary residue had settled in the neckband of her orange Tennessee Vols sweatshirt. Her mother reached over, dislodged a crumb from her daughter's face, and transported the morsel to her own mouth, smacking her lips.

Ruby Lee gently patted her mother's arm. "I'm sorry you can't have no sweets now that you got sugar diabetes, Ma. You know I'd a give you more'n half of this here bun if it wouldn't make you sick."

"I know, girl. It don't make me no never mind." The adoring look bestowed on Ruby Lee broadcasted to the world she was in good hands with this child.

The gate agent announced the pre-board routine for Orlando was about to begin and everyone needing assistance should make their way to the designated area. In addition, all those continuing from Los Angeles could re-board at any time.

"Sonny's not gonna make it," Ruby Lee wailed to her mother. "I tole him he wadn't gonna have enough time if'n he stayed outside to grab one last smoke, but it waren't about to change his mind. Sonny's always wanted to see Mickey Mouse up close. What if he don't git here in time?"

Her mother was unconcerned. "Hell if I care, Ruby Lee. That brother of yourn ain't never been nowhere on time in his whole life and if he don't git here, we'll jist leave without him 'cause I may die myself afore I git to Disney World, and I shore ain't gonna wait in this here airport for him."

The gate attendant lifted the oxygen tank onto Ma's lap and began to trundle her down the ramp towards the waiting plane. Ruby Lee followed them, stopping frequently to look back over her shoulder for her brother. With no sighting, she trailed the attendant through the jet way towards the cabin and helped ease her mother out of the wheelchair into the middle of the first row of seats behind the bulkhead. Carroll waited beside the door while the gate agent removed the wheelchair from the cabin, and then watched as Ruby Lee patted her mother in place. A blonde girl of about eight, sporting a prominent tag around her neck signaling she was an unaccompanied minor, was already seated in the window seat.

"Sonny's gonna have to sit with furriners and Yankees," Ruby Lee whispered loudly, surveying her surroundings.

"Hell, girl, your travel agent done told you Sonny couldn't sit in our row. That boy's got the nerve of a brass monkey. He ain't never met a stranger and he's damn near forty-five years old. I thank he can manage, now set yoreself down." Ruby Lee did not look convinced.

Carroll made her way into the cabin past the seated pair, glancing down at the top of their heads, again amazed that Nashville fashion in 1992 included these crocheted cloches, and then she moved on down the aisle to row eleven. Her seatmate from the Los Angeles flight segment still occupied the window seat while the middle seat remained empty. She slid into her aisle seat and closed her eyes waiting for everyone else to board.

When there seemed to be a lull in activity, she opened her eyes and leaned a little to the left to confirm the end of the line of arriving passengers. Hearing the flight attendant announce she was about to close the cabin door, Carroll let out a little sigh of relief. *If Sonny made the flight, looks like he won't be seated next to me*, she thought. She buckled up, pulled her glasses from her purse, and began to flip through the pages of the professional journal she had already studied on the first segment of the flight.

The odor of tobacco was the first thing to hit Carroll as the man approached row eleven. She had awakened every morning of her childhood to the smell of an unfiltered Camel cigarette—the first of two packs her father would inhale before bedtime. Carroll shuddered as she recalled a recent conversation with Jeanine, her closest associate at work.

The two women had been enjoying a rare after-hours drink on the patio of Batson's, a small bistro near their Los Angeles office when a well-dressed twenty-something woman lit up at the next table. Speaking more loudly than usual, Carroll told Jeanine, "I hope it won't be long before the rest of California does what Beverly Hills and San Luis Obispo have done. At least they had the guts to put a complete smoking ban in place. It's insane—just insane—the way we're all exposed to second-hand smoke everywhere we go."

"Well, I'm sure as always you'll be a one-woman team campaigning for the law to be changed," Jeanine said, laughing and raising her wine glass in salute to her office mate and friend. "After all, you don't have anything else on your plate."

The two women laughed and Carroll raised her wine glass, accepting the good-natured jibe.

"I know—I am a bit of a crusader some times. But I just can't stand to see things that need to be righted and no one seems to do anything about them."

"Did you ever smoke?" Jeanine asked. "I know I did—everybody did when we were in college."

"No, I couldn't stand to be around cigarettes ever in my life," Carroll spit out. "Early on I didn't have much choice, though. I worked in bars and restaurants to pay my way through college, and after all the smoke I inhaled there, I'm surprised I don't have cancer today."

Her voice thickened and she looked down at her hands, pausing to compose herself before adding, "Smoking killed my dad when he was barely thirty."

Carroll felt her inner emotional corset threaten to relax, and then she pulled the lacings tight and the moment passed. Continuing, she added quietly, "And I imagine by now it's also killed my mother."

Jeanine continued, "I've never heard you mention your undergraduate days. Where did you go?"

Carroll swirled her wine glass, watching the legs ascend then slowly retreat into the fluid still in its bowl. She took another sip before answering.

"Warfield for the first semester, and then I transferred to the University of Oregon and that's where I graduated."

Jeanine sat back in her chair and looked directly at Carroll. "Warfield?" she said. "I would never have taken you for a Warfield coed. I thought you were from Chicago. How did you get to Warfield?"

Carroll breathed in, then letting it out slowly, she said, "It's a long story."

She felt her heart skip a beat, and then she quickly shifted in her chair and raised her glass to her friend before tilting the remaining fluid into her mouth. After swallowing, she endorsed, "Here's to a total ban on tobacco everywhere in the world."

The woman who was smoking turned and exhaled in the direction of their table, and Carroll stood up, grimacing, and signaled Jeanine that she was leaving.

"Gotta run, but just you wait," Carroll said under her breath as she fumbled in her purse for cash to leave on the table. "A smoking ban will happen and then we'll see who the winner is."

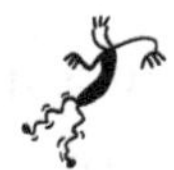

As the tobacco odor in the airplane cabin grew stronger, Carroll looked up over the rims of her reading glasses and noticed the rotund shape and unkempt beard of a man who had to be Ruby Lee's brother maneuvering his portly self down the center aisle. She noticed he was slowing at each row and looking carefully at his boarding pass with squinty eyes, as he got closer to row eleven. Above the tattered bill of his cap was an endorsement for *Bruton Snuff.*

I knew it, Carroll thought, as she heard the man ask, "Id dat my place?" He was pointing his yellowed finger to the middle seat. Carroll turned her head up and saw a gap-toothed grin that somehow managed to escape from under his unruly moustache. With reluctance, she acknowledged the emptiness of the space and stood to let him enter.

"Sonny's the name," he volunteered extending his rough, stained hand to Carroll, who lamely shook it. "I ain't never been on no aero-plane before, honey. How 'bout you?"

Carroll cringed—she'd hated being called honey since she was a child—and she glanced sideways at the other woman, who rolled her eyes and pulled out her book to read. Sonny rubbed his hands on the ragged, torn knees of his jeans and tugged at the hem of his plaid flannel shirt in an attempt to get it to cover his ample belly, to little avail. The flight attendant leaned in and reminded him to buckle his seat belt, handing him an extension piece.

Sonny turned to the woman on his right, "I drive a truck for Metro," he volunteered. "Been there damn near six year."

His window seatmate had now drawn herself into the glass pane of the porthole, so he turned his attention back to Carroll. Pushing the bill of his cap back away from his face a little, he turned to his new potential friend on the left. "So, what you do for a living, honey?" he asked, reaching over to pat her on the knee.

Carroll drew in her breath. She covered his fleshy paw with her well-manicured hand and lifted the offensive limb from her leg. Straining against her restrictive seat belt, Carroll pulled herself up to the tallest position she could manage and leaned over into Sonny's space, then gazed down at his crotch with a hard stare.

She could feel her amber eyes glisten and her fiery red hair felt electrified. "I'm a sex therapist," she replied, sucking in the remainder of her breath through clenched teeth, "and I can tell by looking, you definitely do not measure up."

Satisfied that she had pushed back Sonny's overture, she reached for her medical journal and read for the rest of the flight. A couple hours later, after the plane landed in Orlando that Thursday evening, Carroll hailed a hotel shuttle. As she boarded the van, she heard her name being called from the back row of seats. She searched through the dark interior and located Maria Grayson, one of her long-time colleagues in the professional world of sex therapy.

"Hey, Maria, good to see you, How are you?" she asked.

"Fine. Come on back and sit here, Carroll. I guess we're both going to the same conference, huh?" replied Maria.

"Yep, gotta keep up those continuing ed credits somehow."

Both women laughed.

"How've you been? My clients are always telling me about what they've heard you say on some TV show or I'm reading about you publishing some new breakthrough book, but I haven't actually talked to you in ages," Maria continued.

"Oh, Maria. I've been crazy busy—mostly it's all good. However, at the moment I think I'm in shock. You are not going to believe what I just said to someone on the plane coming here. I have never in my life allowed anyone to get under my skin like this, but something about this guy got to me and I just cut loose on him. I feel really embarrassed—it was definitely not the me the public sees on TV."

"I can't wait to hear about it—some poor shmuck got to the world's most famous sex lady. That should be good for lots of laughs at this conference and later, my friend."

"I'm afraid you're right, Maria," Carroll said, shaking her head and grinning as the van pulled up to the hotel entrance.

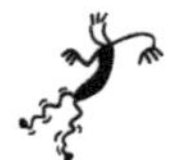

PART TWO: SEX and DANCING

Sunday, August 16, 1998

Dulles Airport, Virginia

Carroll dropped into one of the few seats still empty in the waiting area and audibly sighed at her bad luck. *Déjà vu, all over again*, she thought, glancing at her ticket from Washington to Los Angeles via Nashville. She unleashed her shoulder-length mane of auburn hair from its decorative clip. Resting her glasses on her thigh and leaning over so her hair could fall forward, she grasped the unruly tresses and attempted to rewind them into a knot at the back of her head.

"Shit," she muttered and again cursed her inheritance of the Murphy curly hair, which had been her lifelong nemesis. Hair and airline schedules were about the only parts of a tightly managed life over which Carroll had not been able to gain control.

"There must be something you can do. I absolutely refuse to be routed through Nashville," she had pleaded, first on the phone with her travel agent and then with the gate agent. *If I didn't have to be in L.A. for tomorrow's schedule, I'd fly directly to Chicago from here and not have to stop in that place*, she had thought. *The show gives me such short notice!*

In the six years since her encounter with Sonny en route to Orlando, Carroll had traveled thousands of miles, but she had never been back through Tennessee's capital city. *Everybody in that city is either a redneck or a fraud*, she would remind herself, telling no one, least of all herself, the real reason why she refused to breathe Music City air.

"No, ma'am, sorry. All direct flights are full. The only way I can get you to LAX at this late hour is through BNA."

Even after this long a time, Carroll flinched as Sonny's possum grin flashed in her mind's eye. She let a small chuckle escape as she remembered his exit from the center seat over her legs. As he had worked his way toward the back of the plane, she'd stood for a moment in the aisle to watch his retreat, smiling along with the other female passengers nearby who were silently applauding her. The crimson glow from the back of Sonny's neck verified she had hit her target dead-on in one of the few times in her professional life that she had used her position to her own advantage.

Poor fellow, she thought, shaking her head. *Probably hasn't had a hard-on in the last six years.*

Despite the brief humor this memory brought, Carroll dreaded another airplane encounter with a native Southerner. Reluctantly, she began to observe two attractively dressed women she guessed to be in their mid-fifties who were engaged in a very animated conversation. She couldn't help but notice the crown of platinum hair worn by the taller and more slender of the two women. *I guess it's not exactly big hair but it sure is bouffant,* Carroll thought.

The other woman, slightly younger, was about twenty pounds heavier and an inch or two shorter than her traveling companion.

It'll be just my luck to be seated between them, Carroll thought, reaching into her briefcase for a professional journal to distract her until time for boarding.

Surprising herself, she glanced at them again. It was hard not to notice them. While they did not physically resemble each other, there was something about their eyes that made her think they might have come, if not from a common gene pool, then at least from a common life-experience pool. It was not so much the color of their eyes, bright blue in the older and green in the younger woman, as it was an expression that played around the edges when they seemed to have made a mental connection on something they were discussing. Sometimes the more beautiful woman would lean over and pat her companion on the arm, and both would smile.

Carroll had seen this same knowing look emerge time and again at a point in therapy when two people's stories were merging and what had seemed like a solitary experience became, in fact, a mutual process. In her television appearances, Carroll often cited this experience, calling it an "ah-ha of the eyes," confirming that two individuals must not be as alone in the world as they had previously assumed. In that exchange of looks, she would tell her audience, one person begins to step into the other's shoes and see the world through the other's eyes— "empathy" in therapeutic terms.

"You really have to do this—to connect with them—if you're trying to reconcile with somebody," she often advised. Once, from the spectators, a young man's voice said, "That must be what my girlfriend means when she says 'you got it.'" Carroll smiled and nodded to the man, and the viewers applauded him.

When she was traveling or otherwise spending time in crowds of strangers, Carroll played a game of sorts, in which she would make up names for and stories about her fellow travelers just for her own entertainment. As an only child, she had learned early on to entertain herself with her private thoughts and games, and she suspected this little fantasy was not at all unusual. In fact, her training as a psychologist had taught her that such flights of the imagination could even be therapeutic, as long as she kept them completely to herself.

Noticing more closely the stouter of the two women, Carroll thought, *Almost . . . what would you call her?. . . dowdy. OK, matronly. Definitely a Helen*. She mentally named the other woman Blondie.

Helen, wearing a denim pantsuit and carrying a large see-through plastic purse that more nearly resembled a beach bag, seemed to take the lead in conversation, while Blondie contemplated her fingernails and perfected her beauty-queen smile. Blondie's tight-fitting black jeans hugged her curves and a bright pink V-neck sweater left little to imagine as it stretched over her ample bosom. A large rhinestone-embedded cross threatened to fall into Blondie's cleavage if its silver chain should snap, *but it won't fall very far with that shelf underneath,* Carroll thought, chuckling to herself. She watched in amazement as Blondie repeatedly reached into her enormous black handbag, retrieving all manner of paraphernalia, including nail buffers, mouthwash, and an atomizer, which she would pump periodically, sprinkling her neighbors in the process.

Both women wore white canvas Keds with white anklets, neatly turned down. Carroll could not recall ever having seen grown women wearing what she had previously thought was footwear for young girls. *Must be another local fashion statement*, she thought, flashing back momentarily to the orange crocheted cloches on the heads of Ruby Lee and her mother.

Carroll had never really paid much attention to fashion trends. Early in her professional career she had adopted what she often jokingly called her uniform—black or navy trousers, usually with a cuff, sensible low heels in the best brand of shoes she could find, and a sweater twin set, usually in cashmere, with a pearl necklace and simple earrings. In her media training years before, she had been coached always to dress as though she might be interviewed on camera and to avoid sparkling jewelry, like a diamond pendant or large wedding ring, which might be over-sparkly in studio lighting. The last part was easy, since she had not worn a wedding ring for almost thirty years.

Blondie smiled easily and warmly to almost anyone who looked her way—and many were looking her way in the waiting area. Carroll guessed Blondie had often been the center of such attention and Helen was probably used to being almost invisible next to such a stunning beauty. Sometimes Blondie would yawn and then grin self-consciously if she caught the eye of anyone who had seen her. Helen looked like she might have a headache, because she kept holding her head between her hands. Occasionally Helen would also stifle a yawn, which did not seem to slow either of the ladies down in their discussion.

The gate agent called the passengers for boarding, and as Carroll was arranging herself in the window seat, she looked up enough to see Helen begin to slide into the aisle seat. She gritted her teeth. *I knew this would happen to me. Hope they keep their distance better than Sonny did.* Blondie was seated across the aisle from the two of them, and she and Helen chatted freely across the aisle way even as passengers tried to hurry past them.

In the row in front of Carroll an extremely tall young man maneuvered himself in place then partially turned and peered over the seat, looking at Helen and Blondie. Turning all the way around to face Carroll, he arched his eyebrows. His green eyes clearly signaled he saw trouble on his radar, and he sat back around firmly. Even fully seated, the top of his head was visible to Carroll way above the seat back. She heard him mutter about how the tallest person usually gets the bulkhead while the shortest one gets seated in the emergency exit row, and his head shake emphasized his frustration. Next to him, a mom and her toddler son were settling into their places. The child's mom handed him a small bag of Cheerios and bent down to retrieve his sippy cup and favorite toy from the diaper bag. Seeing an opportunity, the toddler stood and faced backwards to look at Carroll and Helen, handing them a sticky handful of his treat through the gap between the seats, giggling as the little o's cascaded down to the floor under their feet. His mom snapped him back in place and strapped him down in his middle seat.

Carroll put on her glasses and started reading her professional journal, hoping any remnants of curiosity she might have had about the two women would be discreetly hidden from them. Despite this attempt to discourage conversation, Helen turned to Carroll, extending her right hand.

"Hi there. I'm Peggy," she drawled, making the name sound longer than its two syllables.

"That's my cousin, Trixie," and she pointed to Blondie across the way, who was giving Carroll her best beauty queen smile and wave.

Carroll shook Peggy's hand and waved back to Trixie, introducing herself as Dr. Carroll Murphy.

"Oh, are you a doctor?" Peggy asked.

"Psychologist," Carroll replied.

"Where have you been to, honey, if I may be so bold?" Trixie asked, bending her head into the aisle and blocking a latecomer who was trying to get to his seat in the rear of the plane. He scowled and Trixie flashed him her Miss America smile, pulling her head back from the aisle for him to pass.

Carroll jolted slightly at the word *honey*, but, recovering her composure, she told them she was returning from the annual convention of sex therapists which had just taken place in the nation's capital.

"Well, honey, did you fix the president?" Trixie asked, giggling. "Lordy, I think he needs a little bit of your help, if I do say so myself."

Peggy glanced sideways at Carroll, wondering if Trixie might be pushing herself just a little bit, but she did not catch any signal from Carroll that Trixie should button up her mouth.

"No," Carroll answered, smiling, "but you're not the first one to tell me he could use some help."

Trixie leaned back across her side of the aisle, sighed, and rested her head on her seat back.

Perking back up after a few moments, she bent again across the aisle and continued, "E.R.—he's my boyfriend—we were talking about politics the other day. You know, that E.R. keeps up with all the current events in his *National Enquirer*. Honey, he is the best-read man I have ever seen, if I do say so myself. Anyway, he said he thought queers were going to take over everything with all of their agendas, and I just looked him straight in the eye and I said, 'Well if you ask me—and I know you didn't but I'm going to say it anyway—I think we're having a crisis in our government right now because of adultery and not because of any gay people' and then I just walked out of the room. Honey, E.R. and me can't seem to agree about much of anything these days since he got that fundamental religion."

She sat back in her seat, gazing at an unknown point near the cabin door. A few more nearly-late travelers wandered onto the plane, looking dazed and wondering where they could stow their belongings in the already crammed overhead bins.

"It's hard sometimes to have a conversation when two people have differences in opinion," Carroll acknowledged.

Peggy and Trixie mulled this over, and then Trixie stage-whispered to Peggy, who tilted almost all the way across from her side of the aisle to hear her.

"Remember when we saw Dr. Carroll, the Sex Lady, on Oprah? That's her. I know it's her."

Trixie winked and pointed an acrylic nail toward Carroll, holding her other hand in front and pretending not to look. Peggy kept her head still but turned her eyes far left to confirm the investigation report and nodded enthusiastically. After waiting for the flight attendant to finish closing the overhead bin above her seat, she leaned back across the aisle to confer with Trixie. They spoke animatedly for a few minutes, and then Trixie leaned her upper body over Peggy towards Carroll and asked loudly over the roar of the engines, "Excuse me, honey, but have you ever been on Oprah?"

The tall man swiveled his head to take in the sighting while the harried mom craned over the top of her seat. Then they both turned back to pay attention as the flight attendant noted that in the event of loss of cabin pressure, moms should put on their own oxygen masks before attending to the needs of their children.

"Yes, I've been on her show several times," Carroll answered.

"I knew it was you, honey," Trixie crowed.

Her husky voice hinted of way too much time spent in smoke-clogged rooms. "I said to Peggy when we first sat down I knew I had either seen you on Oprah or on Rosie."

"I've been on both shows," Carroll responded.

As the flight attendant closed the cabin door and picked up her microphone to announce the final steps before takeoff, Trixie reached under her seat for her purse and asked, "Honey, is it okay with you all if I come over there and sit in the middle between the two of you?"

Without waiting for an answer, she began crawling across Peggy's knees. Carroll quickly grabbed her journal as Peggy stood to make way for Trixie's imminent descent between them. Deflecting Peggy's chagrined look, Trixie just said, "What the heck? A girl only lives once," and by then she was settled in and buckling up.

The plane began its taxi down the runway, and Trixie squeezed her eyes tightly closed and grabbed Peggy's left hand. As soon as they were airborne, she enthusiastically exhaled. "Wheh-wee! Now, honey, I don't mean to say I'm a regular on these here airplanes, but the two or three times that I have been on one, why I always get scared we'll run into a bunch of birds on takeoff and we'll crash. I heard that happened one time, and I sure don't want to be riding on the plane what smacks in to some of them Canadian geese making their way down to Florida."

Settling herself in, Trixie grinned and continued, "The only other famous person I have ever met before right now was Dolly Parton. Well, you can't say I actually met her, but I did bump into her in the mall back home in Nashville. And, honey, I mean I really did bump into her."

Carroll marveled at the way Trixie's words rolled out in a combination of teen-aged giggle and barroom seductiveness.

"I was helping Rainey—she's my mama—maneuver her newfangled four wheeler—honey, they told me down at the medical equipment store it was the Cadillac of walkers, and it for sure is. It is bright red and don't you just know Rainey, why, she got herself a bicycle horn and she had my daddy—that would be Floyd—put it on the handlebars, and she's turned into a senior citizen speed demon. Lord, honey, she just honks and honks at anybody what even dares to get in her way. Well, anyway, we were trying to get some shopping done on a Thursday morning a few months back when we thought the mall would be deserted.

And it was. Deserted, I mean. So I could just about look anywhere I wanted to without worrying whether Rainey would run anybody off the road. And do you know what?"

"No, what?" Carroll answered after a few seconds had passed and it seemed Trixie was expecting the conversation to continue.

"There I was looking in the window of Victoria's Secret, trying to convince Rainey some people really did wear those thong things they keep talking about that Monica woman wearing. Rainey said, 'How could you stand such a thing riding in your crack all day long?' and I was trying to figure that one out for myself. When we turned around to go on to Sears so we could buy Rainey some of her cotton underwear, Rainey bumped her walker right smack into Dolly. And for once she didn't honk that blasted horn, thank the Lord. And, honey, don't you just know Dolly, bless her heart, why she was the nicest person you could've imagined. She was all dressed up in her high heels and her wig and she just smiled that great big old smile of hers and said she hoped Rainey wasn't too shook up from all the bumping. Then she just sashayed off with her little packages in her hands. Boy, I sure wonder if she'd been shopping in that Victoria's Secret store."

With the plane airborne, Carroll felt the seatback in front of her start its descent into her lap, and feelings of entrapment began to rise in her throat. She let the question of Dolly Parton's shopping habits hang until it lost its energy, then she inched her fingers into the seat front pocket where she had stashed her reading material.

Unable to resist the opportunity to converse with a celebrity, Peggy jumped in. "Trixie and I have been to a wedding and family reunion in Northern Virginia. It was just too exciting for the imagination!" Peggy spilled forward.

The way Peggy said Northern Virginia, Carroll thought she might pull out her passport on the spot to prove to her she had

had it stamped when she had crossed the border of a foreign country.

"And guess what?" blurted Trixie.

Before Carroll could start to guess, Trixie rushed on.

"Peggy and I are just about to pee in our panties because we became real triplets over the weekend."

Carroll didn't know whether to encourage the ladies to excuse themselves and use the facilities, or just to sit there and hear them out. She opted for the latter.

"We used to be twins, but now we're—triplets," Peggy continued. Carroll looked at her searchingly. *Triplets* had rolled off Peggy's tongue with a special reverence that reminded Carroll of the way her college roommate, years ago, had talked about sororities.

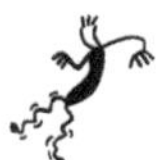

Melinda had come back to their room freshman year after the third round of rush, fairly gushing about her prospects of immediate sisterhood. "Oh, Sunshine," she'd reported to Carroll, as she sprayed herself with Shalimar. "I just love this place. Two dates a night every night for a week and right soon now, I might get to be a real-life Tri-Delt!" As far as Carroll could tell, the only reason Melinda had come to college was to join the best sorority and then to find an eligible male in one of the best fraternities and to get pinned to him.

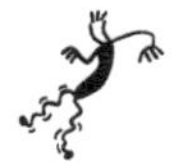

"The two of you are triplets?" Carroll responded.

"Well, I mean there's three of us *now*. We just didn't know we were triplets, though, until we got outed last night," Peggy continued.

Carroll shifted in her seat and began to doubt she would read much of the journal she had opened and closed for the fourth time now. She sighed and slid it in the seatback pocket.

"Now Trixie here, even though she's three years older than me, growing up we pretended we were twins. I was known as the 'Good Twin' and she was the 'Bad Twin.'" Peggy turned and winked at her cousin, before moving her gaze back to Carroll.

Carroll bit her lip before politely saying, "Oh?"

"Honey, it was all because of dancing that we came to be," Trixie intoned with a big roll of her blue eyes, giving Carroll the don't-you-just-know-it look she had seen lots of times on the faces of women whose life experience had begun to match their parents' predictions for them.

"Our mothers always warned us about too much dancing or about dancing with the wrong people, and especially about dancing in loose ways, which could lead to all kinds of trouble for a girl," continued Peggy, looking very serious. Her eyes fixed on the overhead luggage compartment in front of her.

Must be a lot of family baggage there, thought Carroll.

"That doesn't mean," Peggy went on, "I didn't dance as a teenager. *Au contraire!* My parents spent enough money sending me to dance lessons and charm school you'd think I would have amounted to Ginger Rogers after all their effort."

The flight attendant began to explain about unbuckling the seat belts without permission during the flight and about obeying the no-smoking signal. With the seat in front of her now nearly in her lap and the dark blonde hair of the seat's occupant spilling over, Carroll wondered, staring out her porthole, *Can things get any worse?*

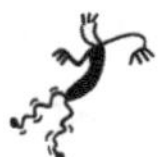

"I'm the second triplet. When I was born, my mama named me Margaret after her best friend, but everybody always just called me Peggy. I tried to get them to call me Margaret when I went to school, since that was the name of that princess in England and nobody was calling *her* Peggy, but it didn't work. Then when I was about ten, that singer, Peggy Lee—have you ever heard of her?—well, she came out with her song 'Fever' and it was on the Hit Parade about a gazillion weeks. You know, when I was little I was sick a lot and my brother, Bobby Gene—he's four years older than me—he heard my parents always talking about my having a fever. So Bobby Gene started walking around playing the strings of his old wooden tennis racket and singing, 'Fever. You give me fever, fever all through the night' every single time I got a sniffle. Since nobody would call me Margaret, I just decided to accept being Peggy. Sometimes I wondered growing up if that darned 'Fever' song would be my motto for life, but I finally grew out of those childhood fevers."

"That's good to hear," Carroll encouraged.

Peggy grinned and her neat row of white teeth caught Carroll off guard. Melinda's Lauren Hutton smile flashed in her mind as she remembered her last look at her freshman roommate.

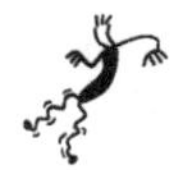

Carroll had stayed in the library until it closed on that cold January night in 1964, her last one ever as a Warfield student, cramming for the Western Civ exam the next day. Making her way across the almost deserted campus towards the freshman residence hall, she found Melinda lying beside a shrub in the frozen grass next to the dorm entrance, passed out and reeking of alcohol and vomit. Her navy pea jacket was open and her sorority pledge pin was partly ripped from her blouse. Her madras skirt was torn at the hem and her stockings were drooping around her knees. Carroll's breath hung in icicles, and at first she thought Melinda might be frozen from exposure to the raw temperatures. As she started tugging on her arm, Melinda moaned, "Please don't tell my sorority. They'd kick me out."

She pulled Melinda up and dragged her into the dorm just before the eleven o'clock official dorm closing time for freshmen, managing to slip unnoticed past the house mother who was involved in helping another inebriated coed get inside. Melinda was still sleeping off her hangover the next morning, a slight smile framing her open mouth. Her tongue threatened to escape from the opening between the teeth, and her arm hung down to the floor. Carroll lifted it back up onto the bed. She considered trying to wake Melinda to say a formal good-bye as she packed all of her things to withdraw from Warfield, but based on her past efforts at home to rouse her mother when she was passed out, she decided it would be hopeless.

Hope you have a good life, Sunshine. Guess that frat boy was not the one for you, so try this pin on for size, she thought. She unclasped the circle pin that was attached to her collar and laid it on the pillow next to Melinda's sleeping head.

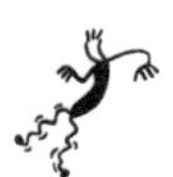

When Carroll rejoined the ladies, Peggy was still talking. "Yes, I became known for my studious nature. I decided at an early age I wanted to go into the medical profession. I guess it was because I had to spend a lot of time in medical offices when I was little with all of those fevers. Now I'm a nurse in a colonoscopy clinic!"

Trying to be heard over the roar of the airplane noise, Trixie practically shouted, "Honey, my second ex-husband, Frank—he was a long-haul truck driver—anyway, he used to tell everybody who would listen that Peggy sees a lot of assholes every day."

The man in the reclined seat rose up and his eyes shot nuclear warheads at Trixie, but they bounced right off. Peggy giggled, blushed, and shifted her weight in the seat. Trying to refocus the conversation, she continued the history lesson.

"Our full name is the Turner Triplets. We're Turners because Turner was my maiden name. Trixie here is my first cousin on my mother's side, in addition to being my triplet sister, so that makes her almost a Turner. I guess it was a good thing she wasn't born on my daddy's side because then she would have been Trix Turner."

The women began to convulse in giggles, and Carroll could tell they had found this play on words immeasurably funny for a long time.

"And guess what else?"

Carroll couldn't even begin to guess what else.

"We discovered we have a third triplet sister named Joan, and she's a Turner by marriage because she's married to my brother."

"That would be Bobby Gene's wife?" Carroll asked.

"The same," Peggy responded.

Carroll's professional brain was in overdrive trying to place all the Turner relatives on a family tree in her head as the women told her their story.

If this group were my clients, by now I'd have their tree in leaf from top to bottom with all these characters, Carroll imagined. *Not to mention all the tentative conclusions I would have reached about this brood.*

Peggy seemed to run out of breath and she reached into her plastic beach bag, bringing out a pack of Juicy Fruit gum. She offered a stick to Carroll, who declined. Pulling out a stick of gum for herself and offering one to Trixie, who accepted with pleasure, Peggy carefully unwrapped the little foil cover and put the gum long ways into her mouth, bending it softly from end to end. She folded the foil neatly into quadrants before putting the wrapper back in her purse. "I might need to spit my gum in it," she explained to Carroll.

Carroll was used to following convoluted stories in her client sessions so she thought she was tracking pretty well, when Trixie dropped the first bombshell.

"Do you know what else?"

"No, what else, Trixie?"

It constantly amazed Carroll the way total strangers would spill their innermost stories in public with almost no provocation. Growing up, she had carefully guarded the secret of her mother's drinking, projecting to the world all was well in the Murphy household. She had managed so well to fool the outside audience that she sometimes even convinced herself things were not as bad as they were. *After all, she is not really an ugly drunk. She just works long hours at the hospital and she has a lot on her mind. And it's hard for her to make ends meet on one paycheck,* Carroll used to tell herself.

"The Turner Triplets is not who we really are," disclosed Trixie, her blue eyes shining.

"Well, who are you really?" Carroll asked, feeling more than a little exasperated.

Peggy glared at Trixie and Trixie shot back a sheepish grin.

"Okay, Miss Smarty Pants. You have already started to let the cat out of the bag, so I guess you might as well tell the rest," sighed Peggy in resignation.

Carroll settled back and stared at her window.

Where is this going? she thought. *And how can I bail out?*

A few weeks back, she had been directing a therapy session between a high-powered Hollywood husband and his new high-maintenance wife, who had discovered he had not been entirely forthcoming before their marriage about his capacity for fidelity. Having heard similar stories many times before, Carroll could almost write the script for what was coming next, and she had begun to drift a bit. Unexpectedly, the wife said, "I've never told this to anyone in my life, but I guess I can tell you here, since we're in Dr. Carroll's office," and then it became *True Confessions* time.

Carroll returned from her reverie. "I'm sorry. What did you say?"

"We are really . . . the Trollop Triplets," Trixie and Peggy said together, letting out a big sigh of relief for having gotten this on the table.

"The Trollop Triplets? That's an interesting name," Carroll said, continuing to give them her best professional manner.

"Yes, well it's sort of a secret name and we have a secret motto and emblem, too," said Peggy, looking a little smug.

"Well, if it's all a big secret, Peggy, then why did you just tell it to a stranger?" chastised Trixie.

"Oh, heck. I guess we can tell a few people, because who knows? There may be some more of our sisters out there."

Carroll's eyes widened in amazement.

"Where did you come up with a name like that?" Carroll asked, conceding she would have to play along for a little bit with wherever this was going.

"Well, as I said a while ago, it started when we were dancing," Peggy said. Trixie's blue eyes began to narrow just a little and Carroll saw the look she'd seen earlier on Peggy.

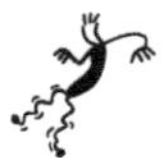

The look. Women can say whole chapters with just a turn of the eye, Carroll thought. As a graduate teaching assistant, she had once considered writing a book on the subject, but she had been discouraged by a faculty mentor who did not think it would be a serious enough topic for legitimate research. Carroll had disagreed with the professor to no avail, remembering vividly that when she was a young child, Frances had been an expert at controlling her by looking at her through slightly narrowed eyelids and just a hint of a pursed mouth. The look said all that was needed to get Carroll to back off anything that might not have fit with her mother's idea of propriety. The same degree of control could be exercised by a clearing of the throat. To this day, whenever Carroll heard an adult clear her throat, she momentarily stopped in her tracks to see if it was a maternal call to order.

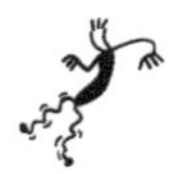

Carroll asked, “Dancing?”

“Yes, you know we told you we are on our way back to Tennessee after being at a big ole wedding and family reunion?”

She nodded.

“It was Trixie’s daughter, Faye, who got married. That girl has really done us proud. After birthing those three rowdy boys of hers, Trixie decided to name her only daughter after that movie star in *Bonnie and Clyde*, which she went to see the night before Faye was born, and it has really paid off. After Faye graduated high school, she went off to college and got herself a job in D.C. and met this boy who was *Somebody* and the rest, as they say, is history. The next thing we knew we were getting real almost-engraved invitations to this and that bridal shower, and Faye was saying she had to have a Vera Wang wedding dress. None of us had ever heard of Vera Wang and we couldn’t see why she would want to go anywhere but Petals and Lace and buy one off the rack because, you know, you’re never going to wear it but that one day, so why spend all your money in one place?”

Carroll pondered this while Peggy went on.

“Well, as I was saying, it had to be a Vera Wang dress, and then Trixie had to have just the right mother-of-the-bride dress, and it had to coordinate with the groom’s mother’s dress, and all such other stuff. Trixie, you tell her what happened next,” Peggy suggested.

“Oh, Lord, honey, I can’t believe it was just last night. There I was as cleaned up as I have ever been, wearing my almost-designer mother-of-the-bride dress—Calvin calls it MOTBD— I had got at the upscale consignment store that I had to drive halfway across Davidson County to get to. My boy, Calvin—he’s my artistic son—he’d done my hair and makeup. You know, honey, he got me a job at the front desk of that fancy salon where he works—it's called the Beautique Salon and Day Spa—and I cannot even afford to step foot past the lobby unless he gets me a gift certificate. Now I am so grateful to have that job since I moved to Nashville because Lord knows I have needed those insurance benefits these past few years. Anyway, he said making me beautiful was his gift to the MOTB. Honey, I am so proud of that boy of mine." Trixie reached over to squeeze Peggy's hand.

"Well, anyway, I had gotten myself strapped into one of those Wonder Bras, and if I do say so myself, it did improve my cleavage. For some time I'd been thinking if I ever did win the lottery—honey, do you know we have to go all the way to the Kentucky line to buy a ticket 'cause they won't let us have a lottery in Tennessee, but Troy—that's Peggy's husband—he drives up there every Friday afternoon and buys us all a ticket—well, anyway, if I ever did win the lottery then just about the first thing I would do would be to get me a tummy tuck or have my turkey wattle nipped, but every time I'd thought there might be an opportunity, Mother Nature would come right along and direct me toward some other kind of surgery. By now I'd had my bladder lifted, my bunions fixed, and my knees replaced, so I was glad to just go to Target and pay $19.99 and get me some cleavage. I mean, most of the womenfolk in our family have natural cleavage when we are young, but after a while it just kindly falls down to our toes and could use a little help, if you know what I mean. Now it wasn't indecent or anything, was it, Peggy?"

Peggy shook her head emphatically no.

"Anyway, I thought I looked as good as I had ever looked, since that time back in high school when I didn't get to go to the junior prom and I already had my dress and shoes bought.

You remember that dress, don't you, Peggy? It's the one we passed down to you after I had Calvin, and your mother altered it so you could wear it to your prom."

Peggy looked nostalgic. "Yes, I remember."

"Anyway, honey, the deal was—even though Faye—she's my little girl—and Mark—that's Faye's fiancé's name—well, he's really her husband now, bless their hearts. Anyway, they were not getting married in a proper church. They were using an old stone house—they referred to it as an estate—and there was a little aisle way what had been set up between the folding chairs. Faye had this funny notion she wanted to be escorted down the aisle by both her mama and her daddy—that would be Frank, my second ex-husband."

Trixie paused to see if Carroll was following her story.

"The long-haul truck driver?" guessed Carroll, as she consulted the family tree in her mind.

"That's the one," Trixie continued. "Well, I thought that was the craziest idea I had ever heard of, since me and Frank did not get along too well when we were married, and we sure as shit—pardon my French—have not seen any reason to keep each other company over the last twenty-five years since we divorced. But after all, it was Faye's big day, so we agreed to bury the hatchet, so to speak, for our little girl's sake.

"Now, honey, this was the first really and truly big-deal wedding I'd ever been in in my whole entire life, since my first marriage to Joe was a quickie across the state line in Ringgold. Then Frank and me got married when we were driving through Vegas on one of his long-haul trips and we'd had just a little too much sampling of those casino drinks." Trixie giggled and shook her head.

"And when E.R.—we call him that because he's a paramedic and he rides the ambulance—when E.R. and I were talking about getting married a few years back, we both just looked at each other and said, 'Been there, done that,' and we moved into his doublewide together."

"I see," Carroll said.

"Anyway, here's what happened. As I said, I was feeling about as good as a girl can feel when she's fifty-five years old and she's got her bladder all tucked up and new knees and her feet don't hurt. I mean, I think I looked *fine*. I walked out to the head of that little aisle way and nasty ole Frank sidled up to me and he said, 'You look like a trollop. Your dress is too damn low-cut and you are spilling out for everybody to see.' It was just vintage Frank. While we were married—which was only about long enough to get Faye started—he always liked to take me out and parade me around town when I got fixed up, and then he'd come home and beat me up because all the guys had been looking at me."

Peggy tucked Trixie's hand into her own and patted it. Carroll could see the sadness that passed between the cousins as they remembered what had triggered this fresh wound. She was grateful the flight attendants were making their way down the aisle taking drink orders.

Peggy picked up the story. "Anyway, I could tell while I watched Trixie going down the aisle, with Faye in between her and Frank, that something awful had happened, because she just looked crushed. I mean, she was still smiling and all, but I've known her long enough to see the pain in her heart, even if she thought she was fooling everybody else, so I couldn't wait to get her alone after the service and find out what had happened."

Peggy's hand rested on Trixie's arm, alternately patting and rubbing her cousin's pain. "Wouldn't you just know it, though—Mark's family was Episcopalian. Faye had wanted to get married in Virginia so all her classy new D.C. friends could be there. Of course, it hurt our feelings right smart for little Faye to not come home to Tennessee to be married, but we decided to not make a fuss about it. If I do say so myself, all of our family looked pretty good up there in that old Virginia estate house. We could hold our own against any uppity Northern Virginians."

"I'll have a white wine, please," Carroll said to the attendant. She held up her three dollars and the attendant thanked her for having the correct change. Trixie looked at Peggy, who shook her head, and they both ordered Diet Cokes.

"As I was saying, it was an Episcopalian ceremony and they had this priest by the name of Father Bob up at the altar. I couldn't believe my ears when he lit into a sermon before he even got around to the 'I do's.' That is just about the tackiest thing I ever heard of, but what can you expect from Episcopalians?"

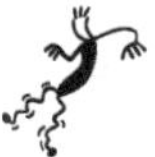

Carroll's last attendance at a church had been during her freshman semester at Warfield. The local congregations sent busses for any college students who wanted to attend services. As a bonus inducement, the students would receive a free lunch afterward. Always practical, Carroll had enjoyed the hospitality of several churches until the Sunday when she was listening to a sermon and the minister declared there was not any basis to think humans were descended from monkeys, and anyone who thought so was a heathen. Already showing her progressive leanings, she had walked out of the sermon and never looked back. A few weeks later, when Melinda and her sorority sisters had donned mantillas and gone as a group to mass, after Kennedy's assassination, she had smirked at their new-found Catholicism. "Religion is the opium of the people," her Western Civ professor had reminded her over coffee. She'd felt emboldened by this Marxist rhetoric.

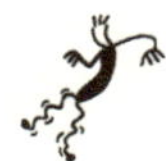

"Tacky? What do you mean?" Carroll asked.

Peggy continued, "Well, growing up, my folks always took Bobby Gene and me to the Baptist church every Sunday morning and evening and on Wednesday nights, unless it was during Little League season. So I saw quite a bit of the inside of churches, you might say. But next to the Catholics, my folks always cautioned me about the peculiar ways of the Episcopalians."

"Like what?" Carroll wondered aloud.

"Well, Daddy always said the Catholics couldn't decide anything for themselves without asking the Pope. If that wasn't bad enough the Catholics could sin all they wanted to Saturday night, but just let Sunday come and they would be right there in that confessional booth getting themselves forgiven, just so they could start all over again with the sinning come Monday."

"But what is it with the Episcopalians?" Carroll asked.

"They drink wine in church!" Peggy's green eyes glinted when she said this, and she turned to see if the effect of this debauchery had sunk in with Carroll.

"Umm," Carroll replied, trying to conceal her amazement that such activity would be offensive to her seatmates.

Like many Californians, Carroll's friends could spend hours looking at Parker wine ratings and cataloguing their own budding wine cellars. Through them, Carroll was beginning to appreciate the subtle differences in Rhône and Burgundy varietals, but she doubted she would ever match their expertise in all things grape. *If I tell them this one they will never let it go,* she mentally noted. *"Quaint," Jeanine will say. "You actually sat through two hours of such nonsense?" Margie will ask me.*

"Come to think of it, I don't see how the little bit of wine they would get out of a communion cup not even half as big as a shot glass could make that much difference, but you should have heard Mama and Daddy going on about how those priests must drink the rest of the bottle themselves after the service," Peggy rattled on.

I probably better not tell these ladies that Episcopalians actually use a common chalice for all communicants, Carroll decided.

"Well anyway, Daddy got mad at the Baptists when I was about thirteen and faster than you could say mud, we were going to the Methodist church, which had all the popular boys, so I guess it was a good choice for me after all, since there sure were some fun times on those Methodist hayrides." Peggy had a faraway look on her face.

"You were describing Trixie and the wedding," Carroll prompted.

"Oh, yeah. I nearly forgot," said Peggy, and she picked up the story.

"So I was sitting there in the family section next to Troy—that's my husband—and wondering if these Episcopalians were going to pass around little cups of wine and when was this sermon going to end, when what do you think that priest said?"

Who knows? Carroll thought.

"He looked Faye and Mark right in the eye and told them to not ever let their marriage get boring in the bedroom, because if that were to happen it might lead to the downfall of the marriage. Can you believe a preacher would say such a thing, especially in public?"

Trixie chimed in, "Honey, if you want my opinion, I think he had already been sampling the wine."

Probably right, Carroll thought, looking at Trixie sideways with a tiny nod of her head.

Peggy continued. "Whatever. Now I have seen some pretty funny weddings in my day because my daddy was a justice of the peace in East Tennessee where I grew up. You could just about expect any two out of four Sunday nights, just as he was sitting down to his sardines and crackers with a hunk of rat cheese on the side and some cold buttermilk, there would come a knock at the front door. And there would stand a bedraggled-looking couple wanting a quickie wedding.

"And Daddy would go get his little black marriage manual and stand that couple up in front of our fireplace and marry them on the spot. Sometimes Bobby Gene and I would be the wedding attendants and sometimes the couple would bring their own attendants with them. Mama always hid out in the back parlor and would not have anything to do with these proceedings. She said she was embarrassed half to death that Daddy did this kind of marrying and besides, she didn't even think they were legal. And another thing, if somebody was in such a hurry to get married, why didn't they just drive another hour to Ringgold and do it there the proper way?

"One time, Daddy couldn't find his black book, so he just made it up as he went along. The bride and groom had been holding hands, and when it came time for him to say 'You may kiss the bride now,' Daddy started waving his finger at their hands and he said, 'You may disconnect now.' I thought Bobby Gene and I were going to split a gut over that. So you can see, I have been to some pretty weird weddings, but nothing topped this one we have just come from."

Peggy sat back and caught her breath.

What'll the next chapter of this saga be? Carroll wondered.

"Well, when I heard what that preacher said about keeping things lively in the bedroom, I stuck my elbow right in Troy's side and whispered, 'Did you hear that?' He looked at me like I had just asked him the $64,000 question and he did not have any clues."

"He hadn't been paying attention, I gather," Carroll said.

"You better believe it. The last time I tried to get Troy to pay attention to anything but his stupid TV, I had to get right in front of it and yell, 'Help! I've just been raped and the kids have been kidnapped!' but even then he just said, 'Baby, you're blocking my view,' so I have quit trying that trick anymore."

"Yes, they say men are from Mars and women are from Venus," Carroll offered.

"Well, I for sure have a Martian for a husband, but we've been married for so long I guess I'll just keep him. I don't want to try to train another one at this stage of the game."

Just then the plane lurched, and Trixie grabbed the arm rests with a look of sheer terror on her face.

"It's a goose," she whispered through pursed lips.

The captain's voice clicked on, along with the seat belt notice, "Uh, ladies and gentlemen, we have encountered a little unexpected turbulence, so I am asking the flight attendants to take their seats and discontinue cabin service at this time. I don't anticipate this lasting long, and we will move around this little bit of weather in a few minutes. Thanks for your attention."

Carroll saw Peggy grab Trixie's hand and together they began praying, "Lord, we just ask, if it is thy will . . . Yea, though I walk through the valley of the shadow of death, I will fear no evil, for thou art with me. Thy rod and thy staff they comfort me. Thou anointest my soul."

Carroll smiled to see how the ladies calmed down. *That's what rituals—either religious or secular ones—do for people,* she would tell her clients.

Seeing Carroll watching them, Trixie shyly said, "Just a little travel insurance to be on the safe side."

"Yes, from the Twenty-third Psalm of the Hebrew bible," Carroll responded.

"No, honey, we were praying from the King James Bible. Now I don't know much about those Hebrews. They may have their own bible, but I do know this psalm came from the Christian one. Church of Christ, to be specific. Brother Royce reads out of it every Sunday morning. First from the Old Testament and then from the New Testament."

Carroll decided not to challenge Trixie's liturgical reasoning. *Backwoods logic. Bet she has never even talked to a Jewish person.*

The turbulence ended about as quickly as it had developed. All three of them were quiet for a couple of minutes, thinking over the midair near-collision with the geese that miraculously had been averted.

Peggy inhaled deeply and shifted in her seat.

When they seemed to be breathing again, Carroll urged, "Going back to the wedding..."

Why did I ask her to go on? Carroll asked herself.

"I thought for sure after the sermon ended they would get on to the ring and the man and wife stuff, but then Father Bob told Faye and Mark to kneel down, and then he started talking real low so the audience couldn't hear, but it looked like he wanted them to take communion right there during their wedding ceremony. And do you know what?"

Carroll barely got her mouth around the now familiar chorus of "No, what?" when Trixie zoomed on with the next stanza.

"Those Episcopalians don't even use little shot glasses. They have one big old goblet and everybody drinks out of it! That is so nasty!" She grimaced.

"Anyway, Faye didn't seem to mind that she might get AIDS or whatever from that big cup, but I was just hoping they wouldn't expect all of us to drink out of it too. And they didn't."

Maybe it's just that Southerners are like what Margaret Mead must have run into in Samoa—living in a world all their own. I can see how she was fascinated, thought Carroll.

"So Faye started kneeling and her maid of honor stepped up to hold her bouquet and to adjust the train on her dress. Now Faye's dress was full-length, but those bridesmaids' dresses just barely covered their you-know-what. The maid of honor bent over to get the train straightened out, and the next thing we knew her whole hiney was flashing the audience! We didn't know whether to laugh or cry, so I just looked down at the floor. I did glance for a second at Troy, and there he was grinning from ear to ear, like he had just seen the newest Playboy centerfold."

Carroll grinned and covered her mouth with her hand. *I can just picture the look on Troy's face.*

"This wedding was getting downright embarrassing, so I started thinking about the wedding present I had bought for Faye and Mark. I wondered if I'd gotten the monogram right on the towels, because it's hard sometimes with these modern weddings where the bride keeps her own last name to know exactly what initial to tell the store to put first and then last and in the middle. And then, do you know what I remembered?"

"No, what did you remember, Peggy?" *Maybe I should just make a flash card with "No, what?" on it*, Carroll considered.

"I remembered when Troy and I got married and we started opening our wedding presents, I couldn't believe my monogram initials spelled Mama's name. That's because Troy's last name is Atkins. And with my first name being Peggy—well, you know, that's what people called me—and my maiden name Turner, there you have it—P, A, T. Of course the A in the middle is bigger than the other two letters, but it spelled PAT for sure. It was bad enough to see Mama's sad-looking face looking back at me in the mirror every time I washed my face, but to add insult to injury, there was her name on the towels whenever I dried myself off. I sure was glad to see those towels wear out."

Add Pat to the Turner family tree, Carroll reminded herself.

Peggy's face brightened a bit as she continued, "I still have the set of monogrammed sheets Trixie's mama and daddy—that would be Uncle Floyd and Rainey—gave us."

"You do?' Trixie looked amazed.

"Yes," Peggy managed a smile." Your mama and daddy must have been consulting with Mama because they gave us twin-bed sheets with PAT monogrammed on them bigger than life. Even today, they're as good as new."

"Peggy," Carroll started, turning to face the source of this tale. "Excuse me for asking this but why do you think Trixie's mother gave you twin-bed sheets for your wedding? Didn't she think you were going to be in the same bed as your husband?"

"Well, I don't really know. But I will tell you one thing. My grandmother was still alive then, and one day about a week before the wedding she took me aside and said, 'Peggy, do you think you're going to sleep with your husband after you're married?' I just about fell over because if she had known that I had *already* slept with him, I guess she'd have died on the spot. But then this is the same grandmother who told my mama she had five children because she'd been raped five times."

"Coming of Age in Appalachia"—I think that will be the next book I write. She could picture the book cover with the Trollop Triplets beaming as they proudly held up the unused monogrammed twin-bed sheets.

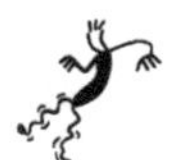

"Ladies and gentlemen, we have come through that little bit of turbulence so I am turning the seat belt sign off. Feel free to move around in the cabin, but we encourage you to stay buckled up while you are seated."

With this piece of news, Trixie raised her hand and said, "Number one," and Peggy instantly gave way for Trixie to vacate the seats. Looking at Carroll, Peggy grinned. "When a girl's gotta go, she's got to go," she chirped.

If I just tell them I need to do some reading, maybe they will leave me alone.

Returning a few minutes later and patting her hands with the paper towel she had brought from the lavatory, Trixie sighed, "The pause that refreshes."

Carroll opened her journal, then shut it again.

"So finally Father Bob finished with the ceremony and pronounced them married, and I thought Troy was going to let out a whoop, but I gave him a look and he pulled himself back just in time. Faye's big brother, Calvin, came over and got Trixie and escorted her out, all the while with Frank glaring at her, but Trixie just raised her head up and never once looked at him, and I was so proud of her."

Peggy squeezed her cousin's hand and they beamed at each other.

"I didn't have much chance to talk to Trixie for a while because they were busy making pictures. I don't know how one photographer can find so many different angles to take of the same scene, but he did. I was standing there watching when he got all of the groomsmen rounded up for a picture of them together. Now I don't often get to see Trixie's three boys—from her first marriage to Joe—all cleaned up at the same time, so I wanted to capture this Kodak moment myself. There they were—Calvin and Walter and Junior—just like stair steps.

"I'll tell you what's the truth," and Peggy turned to her left, facing Carroll and looking across Trixie's face, "when Trixie was having all those boys just one right after the other and she had not much more than turned sixteen herself when Calvin came, I thought all that early motherhood would ruin her looks for sure, but as you can see, she came through just as pretty as ever."

Peggy patted Trixie's bouffant hair and Trixie glowed.

These ladies don't have a mean bone in them, Carroll reflected.

"Anyway, I could see the photographer was puzzled when he was trying to get the boys arranged from shortest to tall, and he kept stopping to look at Junior, Trixie's youngest boy, like he had seen him somewhere before. I laughed to myself because I was sure that photographer would never put two and two together and figure out this boy was the same one whose mug shot he had made in his daytime job with the sheriff's office two weeks earlier, when all of Trixie's people had driven up there for a wedding shower and Junior had gotten himself arrested for stealing hubcaps on Main Street."

"Well, it certainly does sound like it's a small world," Carroll said, laughing despite her best intentions to stay remote.

"Yes, I think so too," Peggy giggled.

"So I decided since it looked like it was going to be a while before I could break Trixie free, I would get a glass of champagne—they said this was the real Brut stuff that costs about ten dollars a bottle, and I certainly did not want to miss out on about my only chance in life to taste some quality alcohol. So with my glass in hand, I walked up to Bobby Gene's wife, Joan. She's the one I was telling you about before—our third triplet. Only I didn't know she was a triplet just yet."

Another branch for the Turner tree, I guess, Carroll thought.

"That Joan surely does have a way of decking herself out and looking like she just stepped off the bandwagon and what she was wearing last night was no exception. I'll bet the total cost of her dress and shoes together must have been more than $100, if it was a penny. Boy, I'd give anything to have clothes like she does, but then Bobby Gene has done real well for himself. He has worked all the way up the corporate ladder to shift captain at the precinct, and that's no small potatoes for a boy who almost didn't finish high school. Why, do you know, one time way back in 1960, when Bobby Gene had just begun riding that squad car, JFK himself came almost through our town on his way to a campaign stop in Knoxville? Wouldn't you know Bobby Gene was the number-two man in the back-up squad car that followed the press car? He almost got to touch the Man himself. Our daddy would have been so happy—he was always for the Democrats even though Kennedy was a Catholic—if he had just lived long enough to see it, rest his soul."

Carroll started to hand Peggy a tissue, but Peggy choked back her sniffle and started in again before Carroll could act.

"So I was chatting up Joan, who, even though she and Bobby Gene have been married for almost five years, I still didn't know very well. He had met her when he went to the police officers' national convention in Detroit, and she was there attending the state teachers' meetings in the same hotel. He said he got on the same elevator with Joan and took one look at her and it was love at first sight. The trouble was, he didn't tell her right then, and when she got off on a different floor than his, he thought he might never see her again, so he went down and rounded up some of his fellow cops and they proceeded to have a manhunt—or I guess you would call it a woman hunt—right in the middle of their convention. Anyway, they found her, and she didn't even know she'd been lost and then, lo and behold the next thing we knew they were married."

The toddler in front of them had escaped his seat belt and stood now, flirting across the seat back at the potential adoptive grandmothers. Trixie reached up and squeezed his sticky hand, and he squealed with delight. His mother promptly sat him back down, shushing his cries and advising him loudly, "Don't talk to strangers."

"Well, I never . . ." Trixie mouthed to Peggy, who just shook her head in surprise at Trixie's being so misperceived.

"So you and Joan were beginning to get better acquainted?" Carroll prompted, despite her better judgment.

"Yes, because, you know, we'd hardly ever been in the same place at the same time with her in the past five years. I'd heard some of the women in the family say they thought she was a little odd and uppity, and being from the north, that would make a person different, with all that snow and hardly any daylight from October until March, but I like to make up my mind in person about somebody. You know the old saying, 'Don't judge a book by its cover.'"

Oh, yes! I know that one well, Carroll thought. She had experienced a lifetime of being judged by the cover because of the spelling of her name. "C-a-r-r-o-l-l is the way boys spell it," her junior-high math teacher had told her when she was grouped with the boys in the assigned seating. In graduate school she had almost been rejected for admission, based on the gender quota system in place at the time. Luckily, she turned up female in person and the administrators were able to change their decision and let her in.

"So I said, 'Joan, I didn't know you had a son as old as Faye.' And Joan answered, 'Yes, I had Richard in my junior year of college. His daddy was playing in the Rose Bowl that year, so we got married on Christmas Eve just before he left for the big game. On New Year's Day I sat there at home watching the parade on TV, and when I saw those Rose Bowl princesses and their queen roll along on their float, I just started bawling. I thought my life was over. I delivered Richard five months later on the very day his daddy graduated. We never had much of a chance at marriage, and we were divorced by the time Richard was two years old.'"

Richard—another bud on the tree—but what was Joan's first husband's name before he was pruned?

"Well, that was a big piece of information, if I do say so myself. Joan went on to say, 'It was a big deal back then if a girl got pregnant before she was married. When my sorority got wind of my condition, they sent me a letter inviting me to turn in my membership pin to the national office because there was no place in their sisterhood for a girl who disgraces their name in such a way.' Now you could have pushed me over with a feather when Joan just came out and told me practically her whole life history right on the spot, but of course it did not change in any way the affection I felt for her."

"It must have meant a lot to Joan to see you were so compassionate," Carroll volunteered, tearing up a little.

What is it about these women that keeps hooking me back in? Carroll wondered. *I'll have to bring this up in supervision with Dr. S. tomorrow when I meet with him.*

"Well, I just couldn't see the point of being in a sisterhood and then when the first little thing what comes along that seems like it would soil their name, they drop you. What are sisters for anyway, if not to hang in there with you and support you when you get in trouble? It just made me so mad to hear what those nasty girls had done to Joan. I began to see why she had kept a little distance between herself and the other women in our family."

Carroll nodded and blotted her eyes. *It does seem pretty unsister-like, I guess.*

"So did you ever get a chance to talk to Trixie at the wedding?" Carroll asked.

Peggy brightened. "Yes, here's the good part. After the pictures were over, they had a big buffet . . . now Trixie, I know you won't mind my saying this." Trixie shook her head, signaling her agreement with further secret-telling. "Anyway, Mark's family had offered to pick up the whole tab, because goodness knows Faye's family couldn't have put on a spread like that. All of us ate ourselves crazy. They had a big punch bowl full of shrimp, and you should have seen Junior. He stood there by that bowl for two whole hours helping himself. He said he figured he must have eaten about $175 worth of shrimp, based on what it costs for a shrimp cocktail at Shoney's, where he busses tables back home. And I reckon he was probably right. Then on top of all that, they had two kinds of wedding cake—one for the bride and one for the groom. And do you know what his cake looked like?"

"Nothing would surprise me," Carroll responded.

"Well, I didn't even know what it was when I saw the danged thing. And then they said it was an armadillo!"

Turning to face Trixie squarely and placing her hand on her cousin's, Peggy continued, "Now, no offense intended for your new son-in-law, Trixie, but if that's not the craziest thing in the whole wide world. I guess that's how they do things in Northern Virginia," sighed Peggy.

"No, honey, that's okay. I thought it was pretty weird myself, but I would not for all the tea in China have said anything about it and hurt Faye's feelings on her wedding day," Trixie answered, patting Peggy's arm.

"Well anyway, after all that eating and drinking about a million toasts to the bride and groom, the band started to play, and right off the bat Mark took Faye out on the dance floor, and they showed off as best they could with him in a tux and her in her Vera Wang dress. They looked pretty stiff, but you could tell they had been to a few Arthur Murray classes. I think they were kind of glad when other people got up to dance so they wouldn't have to be in the spotlight."

Carroll nodded.

"About that time I finally motioned for Trixie to come over and sit at our family table. Up until then she had been sitting at the wedding party table, right next to Frank, because that's where the place card had said she was supposed to sit, but I figured she'd about had it with being proper."

"Honey, I could not wait to tell Peggy what Frank had said," Trixie began. "After we finished all those wedding toasts, I grabbed her and we went to the little girls' room and I asked Peggy what a trollop is. When she told me, I sat down in a stall and cried my eyes out because I have never in my life collected even one penny from anybody because of putting out. But then I had to blow my nose and fluff myself up and come out and put on a front for Faye's sake, but my heart just wasn't in it. I guess Peggy was trying to cheer me up, so she told me what Joan had told her, and then we looked at each other amazed and plastered our smiles back on our faces, and I took her hand and we marched out of that john like nothing had happened.

"And that's when I heard the band crank up 'Rocky Top.' Now of course I stood right up, but hardly anybody else except for our family was standing. I guess those Northern Virginia people don't even know what 'Rocky Top' means."

"What does it mean, Trixie?" Carroll asked.

Both Peggy and Trixie shot her an incredulous look.

"It means you have to start clogging!" they said in unison.

"Or some of us buck dance instead of clogging, but it's all the same—just old-time mountain dancing," Peggy explained.

"Honey, nobody can flat-foot dance and be unhappy at the same time," said Trixie. "So Peggy grabbed my hand, and right away we started therapy for my broken heart."

Carroll inwardly shook, feeling a fluttering sensation along her spine. When she would shiver as a child, her grandmother would tell her "a possum just ran over your grave." She felt tears well up, but she bit her lip and held her breath until they receded. Smiling outwardly, she turned back to her seatmates, where Peggy was continuing the narrative.

"And before you knew it, we had an audience and people were standing on chairs to see us. Even Faye, who in her teens had started to be embarrassed to see us get up and dance even though she'd clogged when she was a little girl, pretty soon she was dragging Mark out onto the dance floor, and there they were—her in her Vera Wang and him in his tux and then almost all the bridesmaids—even the one who had flashed us—trying to figure out what we were doing with our feet. Course, Lisa Marie, my little girl who was one of the bridesmaids, she knew how to buck dance, and she just right there and then started in, and then everybody else got up and tried it."

"But the real kicker was that Trixie and me saw Joan standing over at the edge of the floor tapping her feet, and without even discussing it, we looked at each other and pulled her onto the floor. And she could do it! Who would have known a Yankee could buck dance! And then Troy was out there—and you should have seen him go at it. For a man whose only form of exercise in the past ten years has been to get in and out of his golf cart while swigging a beer and smoking a cigar, that man can still flat-foot."

"Do you know what Troy's idea of yard work is?" Trixie asked of no one in particular.

"Tell me, Trix," Carroll said, exhaling.

Did I just call her "Trix?" Even with her small circle of friends back in L.A., Carroll was never one to let down her guard in such a girly way.

Dr. Sutton probably will say it's transference.

"You tell her," Trixie urged.

Peggy giggled and threw up her hands.

The seat in front of Carroll suddenly bolted forward as the tall man straightened himself up and turned to face Peggy. Carroll could see the resigned shaking of his head above the top of the seat. He hit the flight attendant call button overhead.

Unperturbed, Peggy rambled on. "Well, a couple of weeks ago I noticed some big rocks in our front yard where we couldn't get the grass to grow, so I asked Troy if he would take care of them when he came in from his golf game. He said, 'Sure, Baby,' and that really surprised me, because it is almost impossible to get him to do any kind of work outside in the yard—says it's bad for his allergies, but if that's such a big deal, how come he can ride himself all over every golf course in the county when the pollen count is over two million, and then he can't even stick his fanny out the door when he comes home because it might start him sneezing?"

Carroll could see this was a sore spot for Peggy.

"Anyway, so Troy said, 'Baby, I've got to go to Home Depot to get what I need for those rocks,' and he loaded Spot—that's his bird dog—in the back of his pickup and I figured he would be coming home with a new shovel or something. Well, about thirty minutes later they came back with Troy grinning from ear to ear, and Spot was wagging his tail to beat the band. Troy said, 'Those rocks are fixed for good.' I figured I had better go see how it looked, so I walked out there and do you know what that man had done?'

"No, what, Peggy?"

"He had gotten himself a can of green spray paint and painted those rocks to match the color of the grass."

Jeanine and Margie will laugh me right out of L.A. if I tell them I sat through this entire tale. Carroll shut her eyes, rolling them under her lids.

"The man is hopeless!" Peggy slapped her knees.

The flight attendant brought a pillow to the man, who then reclined again, casting a look of sympathy and resignation to Carroll. Carroll tried to shift a little in her seat, but with his head approaching her chest and Trixie and Peggy filling up the side space, the only place to go was out the window, which Carroll found herself seriously contemplating.

"Anyway, when the band finished the third round of 'Rocky Top,' I finally had to sit down," said Trixie. "I said, 'Peggy, you know I got my bladder tacked up five years ago and then I got my new knees two years ago, and I might ought to take it a little easy. I know all my body parts are under warranty, but I still have to be a little careful.'"

Peggy continued the story. "So we sat down, Trixie and Joan and me, and we all felt so happy. It feels so good just to be with people who love you and who you can be yourself with, and while Trixie was getting her breath and putting ice on her new knees, I told Joan what had happened to Trixie just before she started down the aisle. Joan looked for a minute like she was going to get up and go choke Frank, but she just sat there quietly."

Inwardly Carroll felt herself shaking. Staring out her porthole, she breathed slowly and deeply until she recovered her composure.

"That must have been hard for Joan to hear, given what she had been through herself," Carroll empathized.

Peggy nodded. "Then do you know what Joan said?"

Without waiting for the required response, Trixie rushed on. "Joan said she thought Frank must have graduated from the Redneck College of Sex, to say something like that. Well, honey, that was a real surprise to me because in my time together with Frank—and I will admit it was a brief time—I never heard him so much as mention any kind of education beyond the local diesel college."

"I think I once met another graduate of that school," laughed Carroll, mentally picturing Sonny and Frank together in their robes during the commencement ceremonies at the Redneck College of Sex.

Come to think of it, there might be some other clandestine Redneck College grads I can also name.

Rejoining the girls in their story, she heard Trixie continue, "And I had hardly had time to take in the possibility of Frank's being a double college graduate before, wouldn't you know? Here came old Father Bob with a glint in his eye and holding out his hand for me to dance with him. Not wanting to offend any of Faye's new relations by acting stuck-up, I put my ice bags back on the table and went out on that dance floor with Father Bob."

"And the next thing we knew, they were dipping and swirling. He was a regular Fred Astaire," said Peggy with admiration. "I guess he didn't think things ought to get too boring on the dance floor either," she said.

"I still think he had been sampling the wine," said Trixie.

"Could be," Carroll agreed.

"Anyway, I started looking around for Mr. Twinkle Toes Troy, but he said he was plumb wore out from all that 'Rocky Top' stuff and he would have to sit this one out. So I motioned for Joan to join me, knowing as I did ever since Bobby Gene had his prostate gland surgery he doesn't like to dance fast, since sometimes he leaks a little, if you know what I mean. So Joan didn't want to pressure him if it meant he might puddle in his shoes, and I respect her for that.

"And do you know, Joan can really shake her bootie! I was really surprised to see a girl who spends all her time down in the floor bandaging the knees of five-year-olds in the school where she teaches being able to move so well. But I guess, growing up in Motown, she must have almost known the Supremes and some of those other moving girls.

"So pretty soon we had a conga line going, and then five of those six bridesmaids were shaking their booties, too, and Faye and Mark and all of Mark's fraternity brothers were moving. And even Trixie's boys Calvin and Junior joined in. When I asked them where their brother, Walter, was they said the last they saw of him, he was getting laid by one of the bridesmaids in the limo outside. Now I don't know whether or not this was true, but I wouldn't doubt it. Of all Trixie's boys, Walter most takes after his daddy, and Joe was sure a lady's man."

Peggy nudged Trixie in the ribs and they both rolled their eyes. Carroll was thankful just to shut hers for a moment.

Across the aisle from where the three women sat, in Trixie's former seat, a man in his mid-sixties dressed in business casual wear had been working on a stack of papers. Standing and stretching his over-six-foot frame, he placed the papers back into his briefcase in the overhead bin. Looking across at Carroll, who briefly made exasperated eye contact, he grinned and twirled his finger in a circular motion beside his right ear, then pointed discreetly at Trixie and Peggy. Just as his finger was receding, Trixie looked over and flashed him her beauty-queen smile. Somewhat red-faced he slunk into his seat, but continued to shake his head and grin after receiving a sympathetic look from Carroll.

"Anyway, that party went on until the band quit playing at one A.M. I thought all of us would just fall into bed, but we girls were so wound up we just told Troy and Bobby Gene to go on to bed without us, and Joan and me and Trixie headed for Trixie's room. I think Trixie already mentioned that E.R. couldn't trade off his shift on the ambulance to be there, even though this was the biggest day of the year for Trixie, so to speak. But Trixie didn't hold that against him, because she is just so glad to have finally found a man who has something else on his mind besides tits and ass, she will forgive E.R. for just about anything. Anyway, Trixie had a room all to herself and we three just decided to move in with her for the night."

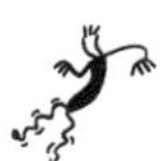

The flight attendant was moving up the aisle with a plastic bag to collect the trash, so Carroll passed her empty plastic cup to Trixie, who handed it to the attendant, patting her hand in the process. "You all are just too sweet, honey. I think this is about the best airplane I have ever been on." The flight attendant nodded and kept moving.

A strong odor of messy diaper began to permeate the cabin in their vicinity, and the young mom shyly looked around to assess the situation. Knowing she could not easily lay her toddler down in the seat to change him without dislodging the man in the window seat, she tapped him on the shoulder. Startled awake, he bounced the reclined seat upright. Only a few seconds contact with the odor convinced him he should abandon his seat while repairs were being made, so he clambered over mom and baby and headed to the back of the plane.

Carroll was grateful she had held onto the napkin from her wine, which she now crumpled under her nose. Trixie pulled out the atomizer. Having spent years working in the colonoscopy clinic, Peggy was completely desensitized to smells of human waste, so she continued with her story unfazed.

"We stayed up all last night after the wedding talking about what all had happened over the course of the past twenty-four hours. I guess it was sort of like a slumber party but here we were a long way from being teenagers but acting just like fifteen-year-olds again. And we popped popcorn in the microwave in the motel room, and Trixie even snuck out to the 7-Eleven about four this morning and got a pack of Salem Lights, but not one of us could stand them now. We had all been quit smoking for too long, so we just threw them away. But we did not throw out any of that ten-dollar-a-bottle champagne we managed to bring back to our room! No sirree, we finished every last drop of the stuff! We even ordered orange juice from room service so we could make mimosas for breakfast."

Peggy and Trixie began to giggle again, and Peggy shook her head and winced, pointing to her head.

"And we got Joan to tell us more about trollops, because to tell you the truth, I wasn't quite sure whether it was a compliment or an insult what Frank had said, but I knew for sure the part about Trixie's boobs falling out of her dress and everybody gawking at her had hurt her something awful."

"I guess that would be something awful," Carroll had to agree, smiling.

"So Joan told us about that Hester Prynne woman whose life story Nathan Hawkins wrote about. Joan said they read about her in English class—*The Red Letter* or some such name of book. I guess I missed school on that day, or else that is just something they teach up north," said Trixie.

"Anyway, I guess we'll just have to read that *Red Letter* book someday ourselves for our book club."

Turning to face Carroll directly, Trixie said, "Honey, do you know what? The next time you see Oprah up there in Chicago, you tell her we call ourselves the Music City A-List Book Club!"

You can count on my doing that, Carroll thought.

Trixie sat back and grabbed Peggy's hand. "Lord, ever since my smart cousin here got her college degree last year, I am just so proud of her. And you had better believe on the second Thursday of every month there'll be about fifteen or twenty of us girls—well, we're really women, but we still call ourselves girls—getting together somewhere being all intellectual just like Peggy. Of course, I usually don't get around to actually reading the book of the month, but so far they haven't kicked me out!" She winked at Carroll, who somehow found her little-girl giggle endearing.

"It's not Nathan Hawkins, Trixie. It's Nathaniel Hawthorne," corrected Peggy, mouthing to Carroll, "She's dyslexic."

"Whatever, honey," and Trixie rolled her eyes.

"Anyway, when Joan finished telling us about poor Hester and how the people in her town made her wear that red letter A, Lord, honey, we felt so sorry for Hester and so lucky we had not grown up living in Maine or Wisconsin or wherever it was that people acted that way."

"And then do you know what Joan proposed?" asked Trixie, looking at Carroll awestruck.

"No, Trixie, what did she propose?"

"Joan said, 'I have an idea. Let's form our own sorority and call ourselves the Trollop Triplets.'"

"We looked at her and then at each other, and we just knew life would never be the same for any of us again. And that's how the Trollop Triplets came to be," said Peggy softly, with the same reverence Carroll had heard the first time the word 'triplets' had crossed her lips.

Just then Carroll felt the first of a series of kicks to the back of her seat. Swiveling enough to see over the seat back, she confirmed the presence of a small boy in the window seat, with a slightly older boy in the middle seat and a man in the aisle seat.

What else am I going to have to put up with before this plane lands? she wondered.

"As I was saying," Peggy continued, "we stayed up all night long and by the time the sun started to come up, we had it all figured out. We decided we are almost just like those uppity girls at the university. Except we're better than them in a lot of ways. We're kin to each other, not just some fake group of girls that get to be pretend-sisters because of somebody's name or a recommendation. You have to actually *do* something in order to get to be in our group."

Carroll could tell by the way she emphasized *do* that this was a big part of their connection.

"What is it you have to do to be a member of your sorority, Peggy?" she asked.

Before Peggy could respond, Trixie leaned over and whispered in Carroll's ear. "Here's the deal, honey. The cardinal and only rule of membership in our sisterhood is: you must have been at least six weeks pregnant with your first child at the time you were married for the first time."

Carroll let this soak in a minute, and then she said, "Well, ladies, I'll bet there are thousands of women out in the world who could be in your sisterhood."

"We think so, too, but we may be the only for-sure certified trollops in our family," said Peggy. "Trixie's mother has been tracing our family tree. Ever since that movie about roots came out, Aunt Lorraine—that's Trixie's mother, but we just call her Rainey—has been obsessed with knowing which boat our folks came over on."

The messy diaper odor had been fixed, and the mother, seemingly having forgotten her earlier fear of strangers, asked if Peggy would mind watching the baby for a couple of minutes while she chucked the offensive material in the lavatory trash. Peggy slid out of her seat and leaned over the little boy, who was happily sucking from his sippy cup.

"No, sweetie, I'd be proud to tend him. I've raised two young 'uns of my own and I can't wait until my little girl makes me a grandmother. 'Course I want her to find a good husband and get married first, so it's all legal and such."

Just then, Peggy noticed the woman was obviously pregnant and wearing no wedding ring, and she flushed. The woman shrugged and moved off to complete her chore.

"Hope I didn't hurt her feelings," she mouthed to Trixie.

Returning to her seat, Peggy looked flustered, but Trixie patted her hand and smiled her assurance that no damage was done.

"After all, honey, maybe she's a trollop like us," Trixie giggled.

"Maybe so," Peggy concurred, comforted by the thought.

"A few minutes ago you were speaking about an emblem and motto," prompted Carroll.

Peggy looked at Trixie, who shoved her in the ribs. Peggy looked around to see if anyone else in the nearby seats might be listening in, but all was secure.

Peggy continued, "Like we said, we're a sorority, and we have a pin and special color and motto. Our special color is red. We used it as the color of the three Greek letter T's—*Theta Theta Theta*—to stand for the three founding members—that's us—and also the first letters of our sisterhood name. Joan helped us come up with that part, because neither one of us learned to speak much Greek."

Trixie reached under the seat in front of her and started mining her purse.

"Look, honey, here's my makeshift Trollops pin. It doesn't look like much right now since we used my nail scissors to cut it out of a Kleenex box in our motel room and then we used an old tube of lipstick and an eyebrow pencil to fill it in, but just as soon as we get situated back home, we'll get us a slicked-up version."

She straightened out the bent edges of the prototype and placed it over her heart, smiling into Bert Parks' eyes.

Carroll thought about telling the new initiates that Joan's help was a little off base, since the Greek letter *tau* actually is the equivalent of the English letter T. *Better not. They probably couldn't handle that much info. I kind of like the sound of Theta Theta Theta better than Tau Tau Tau anyway.*

"I guess you could call yourselves Tri-Thetas for short."

"Oh, honey, I like that. Were you ever in a sorority yourself?"

"No, I went through rush my freshman year, but I didn't feel related enough to anyone I met to become a sister."

Carroll knew this was not entirely accurate, but she did not volunteer any more information.

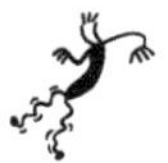

The truth was Carroll had little idea what a sorority was when she entered Warfield University in 1963, but since rush week started right after matriculation, she signed up for it. During the first round of rush parties, she was amazed to see the sorority members dressed up as fairies or angels or honeybees, singing rush songs on the front porches of their sorority houses as the rushees were herded in. Since she had sung the lead role of Liesl in *The Sound of Music* just a few months earlier, she thought maybe she would enjoy this kind of college acting.

I am sixteen going on seventeen. Her clear soprano voice had filled the high school auditorium with its resonance, and her line projection had allowed even the most hard-of-hearing grandmother to understand every word she said. Without her glasses and with her red hair drawn back simply and her stage makeup in place, Carroll shimmered in the stage lights.

Totally unprepared am I to face a world of men, her Liesl had pandered to Rolf, who had already offered, *You need someone older and wiser telling you what to do.*

Bachelor dandies, drinkers of brandies. What do I know of those?

Once, in rehearsals, Carroll had stumbled over these lines, tearing up and taking a quick break into the wings, but within moments she was back on stage, resuming her role. "Never look back," she had heard her father say in her head.

A month shy of her seventeenth birthday, Carroll was already taller than most of the other Warfield freshmen coeds. She wore no makeup, and with her unruly red curls and the thick glasses that had been on her nose since third grade, she was a stark contrast to most of her fellow classmates. She had tried getting contact lenses, but when she was not able to tolerate the hard plastic in her eyes, she had no choice about eyewear. At all the sorority houses she visited during the first round, she was usually assigned to the plainest of the sisters, who took her to a back room and made small talk, while the beautiful and blonde and, most especially, Southern girls were rushed by the more attractive sisters. Once, she had been about to start a conversation with one of the costumed beauties who had shown a spark of interest in her acting background, when the sister noticed Melinda seated a couple of places away. The sister stopped talking to Carroll in mid-sentence, turning to Melinda with a wide smile. "Oh, darling, we are just so honored to have you here with us today and we surely hope we will see lots, lots more of you."

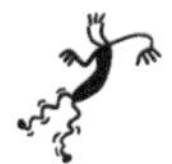

Just then the brother of the four-year-old who had been kicking Carroll began to kick Trixie's seat. Trixie rose up and half-turned, looking at the blue-eyed child. "Honey, please don't kick the seat."

"Don't call me honey. My name is Alexander," he said defiantly. For emphasis, he kicked hard with both feet, while his father smiled helplessly.

Carroll half-smiled in solidarity with Alexander. She had wanted to tell Trixie about a hundred times not to call her *honey* but she'd quickly recognized it would be a waste of her breath.

"If that don't beat all. Nobody ever thinks about telling children no these days," the exasperated Trixie voiced to no one in particular as she rearranged herself in her middle seat. Carroll smiled solicitously and reached over to pat Trixie's hand. Trixie patted back. Together they endured the rear pummeling for several more minutes, until the flight attendant who was patrolling the aisle firmly told the boys to stop, which they promptly did.

"You were saying earlier that you have a motto," encouraged Carroll.

"Yes, our motto is 'We are easy but we are not cheap!'"

They must have come up with that about the same time as they were polishing off the champagne, Carroll thought. *I'd better have another glass of wine if I am going to survive this.* When the flight attendant arrived to take the order, Trixie and Peggy said, after their weekend binge, "Thank you very much, but we'll just have another Diet Coke."

Peggy's history of the Trollop Triplets continued.

"Trixie is the oldest Triplet. Joan says her job is to be the 'Keeper of Wisdom' among the sisters. I could see why Joan would choose this job for Trixie because Trixie had been a big help to me in my growing-up years by explaining to me the facts of life when I was about nine-years-old. At that point in my life I didn't know I was in need of such information, but I suppose Trixie could tell even at that age I was a potential trollop, so she wanted me to be well-educated."

Winking at Carroll, who signaled back with her own wink her understanding of the impending joke, Peggy continued, "Looking back, I can see her intentions were well-placed, but I certainly had difficulty working out what she meant by my gentiles. I just couldn't understand how there were people wandering through the Promised Land—that's what we sometimes called it down there—confronting Israelites and Philistines in my private parts, which I had heretofore been taught to ignore, except when necessary for washing them. Even in those extreme cases, I had been taught I should wash as far down as possible and as far up as possible, and then to wash possible. So how come possible was teeming with gentiles after all that scrubbing?"

Both women laughed at this nonsense tale, before Peggy shifted a little and continued in a slightly more serious vein.

"Anyway, as I was saying, after I got a little older and began to find out the true nature of those gentiles, I wanted to make sure I didn't have any accidents happen to me in the Promised Land that would get in the way of my life plans."

"That sounds like a good idea," Dr. Carroll said, winking back at her again.

Never in her years of practice as a sex therapist had she encountered adult women who referred to their sexual body parts in such unique ways. *Must be something Southern*, she thought, again torn between the intrigue of the story she was being told and annoyance at being held hostage.

"Yes, well, anyway, I figured out right away that the popular form of birth control making the rounds at the time I was entering puberty—namely, after kissing a boy, you drink a

Coke and then you stand on your head—was not likely to work for me because I have never had a sense of balance in situations like that. I thought the scientific approach taught by the Girl Scouts made more sense: you hold an aspirin tightly in place between gripped knees, and that will do the trick. I must say, I became the number-one best aspirin-holder in my class in high school. I even mastered the art of jitterbugging and doing the twist without dropping my aspirin, so you can tell I was really good at this exercise." Peggy's grin gave away the joke.

"You must have been quite an athlete, Peggy," Carroll observed complicitly.

"All this does not mean I hadn't been curious. Those early anatomy lessons held some fascination for me, so I was always glad for the opportunity to go to the local drugstore and look at the latest copy of *National Geographic Magazine* for the photographs of various naked natives, so I could examine their gentiles and other body parts."

Trixie giggled. "Do you remember, Peggy, when we used to spend hours looking at those pictures trying to figure out how they really did the deed?"

Trixie turned to Carroll. "That was after we had about worn out my parents' sex manual that they kept in their bedside table in the Passion Pit."

"Trixie," said Peggy, alarmed. "It's not nice manners to talk about the Passion Pit in public."

Chagrined, Trixie slumped down in her seat and stared at her pearlized fingernails, before continuing.

"Well, honey, if you will remember, we found they had a bookmark after page thirty-two, and all the times we looked at that book, the bookmark never changed places, so if you ask me, I think the reason I never had any brothers or sisters is I was just an accident and after me, they maybe never did it again."

Carroll remembered one of her graduate school faculty had been researching nineteenth-century marriage manuals for his post-doc fellowship. As his teaching assistant, she had spent hours reviewing these historical books, collecting data on courtship and domestic life. She had attended his paper presentation of the topic and later had been pleased to see the paper published in a prestigious journal.

I think I'd better ask him if he has done a phase-two study—sex manuals of the 1960s. I could suggest a couple of new research assistants!

Trixie continued. "Joan, our third sister, is like the mystery sister. Honey, Peggy and I secretly think she was left behind at our conception—sort of like what happens when those test-tube babies get frozen because only one or two are needed right away, and then thirty years later someone looks in the Frigidaire and pulls one out and heats it up in the microwave."

Peggy picked up the story. "Maybe the idea of three Trollop Triplets coming out all at once was just too much for Mother Nature to handle—but Joan somehow found her way back to us this past weekend, and we rejoiced to have her because it can be pretty lonely hanging out in a family like ours where there are no other known trollops."

She patted Trixie's arm, which seemed to revive Trixie's spirits for the moment. Thanks to the second glass of wine, Carroll was feeling a little looser, too, and she added her pat to Peggy's.

"At any rate, Joan's trolloping pedigree was right up there with ours. It didn't take us any longer than it takes to say hello to size her up and to know we were looking at one of our own.

Now as I have already said, some of the other relatives thought she was a little odd because she didn't eat cornbread and could not even get a scald on fried chicken, which everyone knows is the only way to fry it tender and crisp. But none of those qualities matter one bit to Trollops, because, as we have already said and will say as many times as we need to—we are easy but we are not cheap." She and Trixie exchanged a knowing look.

By this time, Carroll recognized her cue, and with their fingers dancing in the air to synchronize, the three of them repeated in harmony, "We are easy but we are not cheap."

That said, Peggy and Trixie withdrew into their private thoughts for a little while, which frankly was fine with Carroll, because she was getting dizzy and she did not think it was from the second drink she had ordered.

With the forward seat again reclined in her lap and the child behind her having resumed kicking the back of her seat, Carroll's prison cell shrank even smaller. She focused her attention on the little red and blue triangle pattern at the edge of the reclined seat and tried to meditate, using *ummm* as her mantra. She was a regular at yoga and almost always could slip into a restful, meditative state with ease after a hectic day of clients and media contacts, but her usually reliable skills could not be summoned on this occasion.

If you can't lick 'em, join 'em, Carroll sighed, and turned her attention back to the ladies with a little smile.

"The thing about Joan, though, that sealed the deal for Trixie and me, was she was a Turner by marriage. She was the real deal!" Trixie chimed in on the last two words.

Carroll nodded her understanding.

Peggy continued, "When we considered the possibility of having an actual in-the-flesh other triplet, at first we kind of liked the sound of The Turner Trollop Triplets. Joan finally convinced us to just stay with being The Trollop Triplets, since it's hard to get all those words that start with T out of our mouths without stumbling over them, so that's that."

Peggy continued the story. "Joan says in our initiation ceremony we can mention the full original name just for the historical significance."

Carroll was glad to see these women had a sense of history.

Trixie chimed in, "And, honey, do you know what else Joan told us? She said she thought we ought to start our first college chapter—she called it colonization—right on the campus of that Redneck College of Sex. Now Joan didn't tell us exactly where that school is located, but she said setting up a chapter there should cause some really big doings, so we're going to talk about it when we get back home and then see what we need to do. "

Just amazing, Carroll marveled.

Trixie continued, "Now, since we just started this whole shebang last night, Rainey doesn't yet know about us—I mean, about the sorority part—but I'll probably tell her one of these days. Come to think of it, she may know some other women in our family who qualify for membership. She's always been right touchy about those marriage and birth dates in the family tree."

While Trixie's wheels were turning, trying to do the math in her head, Peggy picked up the tale.

"From what Rainey—that would be Trixie's mama, she's married to Trixie's daddy, Floyd, who is my mama's brother"—Peggy glanced at Carroll who nodded her understanding of the Turner family tree—"has come up with for the wheres and whens of the clan, the wedding dates before our generation seem to have always been at least nine months before the first little one showed his or her face to the world.

Now, of course, we know that doesn't necessarily mean anything, because in our neck of the woods, there has probably been a fair amount of fibbing on those dates."

Trixie clucked her tongue. "Rainey's always saying about somebody, 'How'd they manage to find a white maternity wedding dress to wear down the aisle?' It just about did her in when my first young 'un, Calvin, put in his appearance in 1960 just six months after me and Joe tied the knot in Ringgold. All poor Rainey could think about then was how was she going to get repaid for all those nice baby gifts she'd given everyone else's daughters, because she was still helping me get my wedding thank-you cards out when I went into labor."

That would be a problem, Carroll reflected.

Peggy continued, "So it doesn't necessarily mean we are the first generation of trollops on the family tree, just the first ones to register our claim to the title. We have learned at least Trixie and I come by our trollop ways through genetic predisposition—"

"She learned that word in college, honey," Trixie interrupted.

"—via our great-uncle Marvin, whose male trolloping eventually drove him out of Tennessee to Texas, where he hid out for the rest of his life.

"And I guess my first ex-husband, Joe, is a natural-born male trollop wannabe, since his daddy made a baby boy out-of-wedlock with one of his organ students while giving her lessons when Joe was in high school," said Trixie.

Peggy giggled. "Joe's family has always had a lot of rhythm, don't you know?" she confided to Carroll, confirming the inside joke with wrinkled eyes and upturned mouth. Carroll muffled her giggle with her napkin.

"Also, Joan reminded us of the fact that all girl trollops must have a boy trollop-maker out there somewhere, in order for a proper trollop event to occur in the first place, so on that score, my husband, Troy, without whose help I would not have had a premature baby, certainly has a claim to auxiliary membership." Peggy continued.

With her college degree, Peggy has a future in the role of protocol manager for this group, Carroll thought.

Trixie looked even more puzzled at these added facts and turned to Peggy.

"What's rhythm got to do with it, honey?" she asked.

By this time they had been in the air for over an hour, and Carroll knew the expected flight time was about two hours. She understood Trixie's doing—or maybe it was her undoing—came when she was a teen in a tryst with Joe and that Joan's actions had occurred while she was in college, but so far Peggy had said little about the circumstances of her doings, other than to mention Troy's involvement.

"Peggy, tell me more about you and Troy," she said.

"Oh, Troy has been the love of my life since I was about sixteen, though sometimes I can't see why I let him stick around for another day with all his crazy ways."

She gazed off into the distance momentarily.

"We were both going with other people when we met," she said. "We were on a high-school bus trip when he first spotted me. I didn't want anything to do with him at that time because I thought all football players were big jerks. Troy was the quarterback on the football team, and I was one of the majorettes for the band, so whenever one of us was going to a ball game, you could pretty much expect the other one would be there too.

"Even though I was two years younger than him, I was only a year behind him in school because he'd had to repeat fourth grade, but we had algebra class together. I think it might have been his third time to take that class, and he knew he had to pass it if he was going to graduate and get to accept a football scholarship to UT—you know, the Vols."

Carroll nodded her understanding.

"Now as I have already said, I was real studious, if you can picture a baton twirler being a bookworm. So algebra was a snap for me, and Troy was always asking me to help him study so he could pass those tests. Just before homecoming I told him he could come over to my house and I would tutor him to get ready for the big test. It was about all I could do to keep his mind on the books, because all he could think about was winning the ball game on Friday night, but I got enough learning shoved into him that he passed with a C-minus, so he was feeling real grateful to me.

"Anyway, he went out and played great and our team won, and afterwards at the homecoming dance he snuck up right behind me when my boyfriend, Delbert, had gone to get us Co-colas, and he slipped his hand around my waist, and my heart started beating so fast I thought I was going to die. I didn't sleep for two whole nights just thinking about what it felt like to have his hand on me, and when I got to school on Monday, I was afraid he would just ignore me because he was such a big deal football player and it was mostly because of him that our team had won, but do you know what?"

"No, what?"

Before Peggy could answer, Trixie butted in and gave more details on Troy and the game.

"Honey, do you know what the newspaper said in its headline in the sports section after that game?'

Carroll was getting more than a little tired of this guessing game, but she echoed again, "No, what?"

Trixie's eyes shone. Pasting the words in the air with her hands, she said, "'Atkins leads team to victory. Does everything on the field but carry the water buckets!'"

Carroll was beginning to be impressed by Troy.

Peggy smiled. "Even though his head could have been swollen to a bushel basket after that kind of publicity, Troy was just as nice to me on Monday as he had been on Friday. Before the day was out, I had taken off Delbert's class ring, which I had wound around and around with strapping tape to make it fit my finger, and Troy had broken up with Mary Sue, and from that day on we have been an item."

Peggy sat back, and for a moment, Carroll thought the plane had lifted up beyond the cloudbank that had blocked the sunshine, because light seemed to radiate off the entire interior.

"Of course, Troy was going off to play football for the Vols in the fall, and I still had another year of high school and then I knew I'd have to work to save up to go to nursing school, so Troy and I didn't make any plans to get married right away."

"I see," responded Carroll.

"Dr. Carroll, can you believe those folks up on the Hill really expected Troy to take a full load of classes and to play football at the same time? They didn't even give him any slack for not being gifted in math," Trixie said indignantly.

"Really?" Carroll played along.

Peggy continued, "Anyway, after flunking freshman math for the third semester and not doing too well in any of his other courses except for P.E., they said they were pulling his scholarship, and that was the end of his football career. To tell you the truth, I was secretly glad, because back then I thought why does a boy need a college education if all he is ever going to do in life anyway is fix up cars in his uncle's body shop?

"By the time I was twenty-one, I was back home newly graduated from nursing school. By then, Troy and I had moved on from hand-holding and lip-locking to some pretty serious making out, but up 'til then we had never got beyond heavy petting with our clothes on. Then one cold December night, Troy and I were at the drive-in movie theater, sitting in his '57 Ford with the engine running so we could keep warm and the windows were all steamed up, and just out of the blue he said to me, 'Peggy, can you sew?'

"Well, I was flabbergasted because he knew I could sew. I had made all my clothes to wear from the time I was in eighth-grade home economics and we had had to sew pajamas and aprons. But as I've already said, Troy is a little on the side of forgetful about certain things, so I guess he just didn't remember, sitting there as we were with not much fresh air in that car and the motor running."

"Before we could hardly get untangled from each other, he went on. ' Look here,' he said, and pointed to his fly. Well, I didn't know what he was about to do, because even though I knew sometimes Troy would get real horny when we'd been making out, he had always respected me. Even after going steady for five years, he had never once forced himself on me. Looking back, I don't know how he managed to keep his sanity because for the last thirty years since we got married, he has tried to do it about every other night, but somehow he did not go crazy back then."

"Maybe he was taking care of himself, honey," said Trixie. "I never was so lucky. Every boy I ever looked at twice from the time my boobs started to grow has just about gone nuts trying to get in my pants. If I heard it once, I heard it a hundred times, how some guy was going to die of blue balls if I didn't somehow get him off before long. And they always said it was my fault and I had no right to just leave them hanging. Being the softhearted person I was, I would always help them out. That's how little Calvin got made, and then Walter, and then Junior. By that time I had figured out what was causing all those babies, and I put a stop to it, but that didn't stop Joe from pestering me, and when I said no, he would just walk out the door and go find him a female companion somewhere else."

What a sad life for a beauty queen, Carroll thought.

Peggy picked up her story. "So Troy is asking me if I can sew and before I could answer, he had started to take off his pants and he said the reason he was asking was because his fly was all torn up and he wondered if I could fix it. So here I am, sitting in the backseat of his car in a drive-in movie in the dead of winter with a man who just has on his jockey shorts, and we started giggling and messing around and then before I hardly knew what was happening we had done the deed!"

Peggy seemed relieved to have gotten this story out, and she signaled the flight attendant she needed another Diet Coke, and Trixie had to have one, too, and so Carroll said sure, she would have one also, since the price was the same for all three. And they all began to giggle.

Peggy excused herself for the trip down the aisle to the forward lavatory. She knew only first-class passengers were supposed to use this one, but the line waiting for the rear toilet was pretty daunting and she was feeling bold. Returning to her seat, Peggy smiled and shook herself out a little before sitting back down to pick up the tale.

"So three weeks go by and the curse hasn't come yet and I pretty much knew I had been knocked up, but I didn't want to tell Troy because even though we had always known we would get married someday, he had never up to that point actually asked me directly to marry him. And I had always wanted to have an old-fashioned, honest-to-goodness wedding with a flower girl and ring bearer and all of that."

Carroll nodded.

"Also, I knew Mama just had her heart set on having a big old photograph of me in my wedding dress to hang up in the front room where all of her friends would see it when they came over. It seemed to be some kind of status symbol that screamed out 'My daughter is a *Nice Girl.*' It just never seemed to be that big a deal to me, but it was to Mama, especially after Trixie didn't make it, and being that Trixie was the only child of Floyd and Rainey, there weren't any more chances for Rainey."

Peggy looked at Trixie and patted her hand. Trixie returned the favor, and then Peggy continued.

"Mama and Rainey were always competing to see which one had the cleanest house or could cook the finest meal or something like that, so even though she would never admit it, Mama had her nose a little bit stuck up in the air after Trixie's sudden marriage, and she was always checking to see if my period had come. She called it falling off the roof. I don't know why she used that term when everybody else I knew called it the curse, but I knew every month or so I would get the question about had I fallen off the roof yet?"

"And you hadn't?" Carroll asked.

"That's right. I figured I must have gotten pregnant that very first time at the drive-in movie. I was sure as could be I was going to have a baby, so I figured it would only be proper to let Troy know so he could make up his mind about whether he wanted to stay or leave.

"So I told him. He looked me right in the eye and said, 'I love you. Will you marry me, Peggy?' And I just fell to pieces that he would treat me so great. We got married on the weekend before Valentine's Day in a little church service with just our families there, and I wore my homemade wedding dress which I had had to alter around the waist a couple of times, but it was one of the happiest days of my life. Mama was pretty much in shock with all that had happened so quickly. Even today with her sitting up there in that nursing home where she lives, we will show her the wedding pictures and she just says she still can't believe I did this to her."

All three ladies sipped their Diet Cokes, swallowing the gist of Peggy's revelation.

"Did you and Troy go on a honeymoon after your wedding, Peggy?" Carroll asked.

"Well, not exactly. I had to work at the clinic on Monday, and Troy had a car that was due out on Tuesday, so we just went back to Troy's apartment. After we had hung up those monogrammed towels I was telling you about and had put away two of the three toasters we had received, we spent the rest of the weekend going back and forth to the K-Mart trying to get dishrags and hampers and all those other necessities we had not received as wedding presents."

"Tell her about your pre-wedding honeymoon, Peggy," urged Trixie.

"Oh, that," and now it was Peggy's turn for the eye rolling. "It was sooo embarrassing," she sighed.

"Sounds interesting to me," Carroll encouraged. For some reason she could not fathom, she was beginning to feel a kinship, if not exactly a fondness for her companions.

So unlike myself, she puzzled.

"Just before the wedding, we were out riding around looking for places we might want to live someday if our ship ever came in, since we couldn't stay in his one-bedroom apartment for too long with little Lisa Marie on the way.

"Lisa Marie—that's what we named our baby girl. Troy was so excited that Elvis and Priscilla's daughter had been born in Memphis the week before we got married, and he told me then if we had a girl we were going to name her Lisa Marie. I told Troy, with her being born right after Elvis and Priscilla's daughter, maybe she ought to have a different name in case people got the two of them confused later on in life, but that Troy—he just loved Elvis, and he wouldn't have any other name but Lisa Marie. He said imitation was the most sincere form of flattery and he did not think Elvis and Priscilla would mind, so why should I? And that was that. It's worked out okay just like Troy said it would, and no one has ever gotten those two girls confused with one another."

"The honeymoon?" Carroll prompted.

"Oh, yeah. Well, anyway, Troy saw this sign advertising a motel room up near Gatlinburg—we all lived in East Tennessee back then, you know. $13.99 for one night with breakfast and a TV included—and he decided right then and there we would go spend a weekend there just as soon as we could, because he told me we were already married anyway in his eyes, so why should we wait until we just had that little bitty piece of paper to make it legal. I said I thought it might be hard to get away from Mama, who was keeping an even-tighter eye on me since that wedding day was right around the corner. She kept asking me about my roof falling-off status, and finally I just fibbed to her and said it had come early and she had missed out on it. I sure didn't want to lie to her, but if I'd told her I was pregnant before the big day I think she might have died of embarrassment. So she played along, even though I think she knew all the time. She always liked to say, when we were going to other weddings, she could sniff out whether this was one of those immaculate conceptions."

"You were saying about the honeymoon," prompted Carroll again, thinking they might be landing in Nashville before she would hear about it.

"So one day about a week or so before we were getting married, Troy and me finally told Mama we were going to visit his cousin Emma down in Chattanooga and might not make it back before dark, so we might decide to spend the night there and not to worry about us. Then we took off toward Emma's for about as long as it took for us to get out of Mama's eyesight, then don't you know, we turned that '57 Ford around right smack dab in the middle of the road and hightailed it to that motel."

"Honey, wait 'til you hear this!" Trixie jabbed Carroll in the ribs, brushing against her lap tray and tipping the remains of the Diet Coke into Carroll's lap.

Carroll withered as the cold liquid ran down between her legs and under her buttocks. Raising up a little above the wet seat, she was grateful to see Trixie pull out a roll of paper towels from her purse and begin to mop Carroll's lap and the armrest. Grabbing a handful of towels, Trixie folded them into a pad and slid them under Carroll's backside.

"Sorry, honey," she smiled sweetly at Carroll, who smiled back gamely. Carroll eased back down in her seat, feeling the damp paper pad and wondering if there was any way out of this situation.

I think I'm doomed to Trollop hell, she concluded, noticing out her window that the lights of a city were coming into close proximity. *Maybe for once, Nashville will provide me with some relief, though.*

Peggy continued. "Well, Troy went and signed himself in while I scrunched way down in the floor of the car so the desk clerk wouldn't see me when he craned his neck out the window. The clerk told Troy he could just park out front and bring his bag in and walk up the front stairs to his room, and he handed Troy the room key.

"In today's times, that may not seem like a very big deal since everybody just shacks up with everybody else at the drop of a hat, but in 1968 it was a very big deal, and sometimes particularly snooty desk clerks were even known to call up the local sheriff's office and report guests on suspicion of cohabitation."

How times have changed, Carroll reflected.

"So Troy got himself all tucked in his room and then he snuck down the back stairs and brought me up there, too. Now we were both pretty horny by then, so we just immediately fell onto the bed and started to go at it, when there was a knock at the door just as loud as could be, and Troy jumped up and pulled on his jockey shorts and said, 'Just a minute. I'm taking a leak.' And then just for emphasis, he stepped into the john and flushed that toilet.

"All the time I was jumping around trying to get my clothes all picked up and figuring out where I could hide, since it wasn't a very big room to begin with. So I jumped in the closet and shut the door. Only it wasn't really a closet like you see today. It was a wardrobe, which was standing on the floor up against the wall. And I was shaking with laughter at the mess we had got ourselves into, and that whole wardrobe was just moving from side to side, and then what do you think happened next?"

Carroll was breathless with anticipation.

"The knocking on the door got louder and louder, and Troy opened the door and in walked that snooty desk clerk. He walked right over to that wardrobe, saying he needed to check and see if there was the right number of pillows for the bed. And he pulled open those two wardrobe doors, and there I was just as naked as a jaybird. He just pretended he had never seen me and turned around and said to Troy, 'Well, I guess you have what you need for the night.' And then he marched himself right back out of the room, and Troy and I just about fell down in the floor laughing."

I can't believe I'm hearing this, Carroll thought, looking sideways at Trixie.

"Tell her the rest, Peggy."

"Well, I didn't think we could get in much more trouble, but then the next morning when Troy went to check out at the front desk, he told me to just wait a few minutes and then come on down the front steps, because since the clerk had already seen me there wasn't much reason to sneak out the back. So here I came to the top of the steps, just walking along like I was Miss Astorbilt, not even paying any attention to that desk clerk. And just as I started down the steps, I could see Troy's hand behind his back waving furiously like he wanted me to make myself invisible. I came down a couple more steps, and then I saw the tan uniform of the sheriff's deputy standing there talking to the desk clerk. And I got so scared I tried to take two steps at a time back up those stairs, and the next thing I knew, I was sliding all the way to the bottom on my rear. I told you earlier I am not the most graceful person in the world, and if I get stressed I just about will fall down if I do anything."

Despite her best efforts to remain composed, Carroll doubled over with mirth at this last revelation, which in her tight surroundings meant turning partway around and leaning her head onto Trixie's shoulder. From this contortion, Carroll finally managed to ask, "What happened next?"

"Nothing," said Peggy, sobering somewhat. "It turns out that deputy was there looking for a couple of convicts who had run away from a road detail, and he just thought the clerk might have seen them. So Troy and I got back in his '57 Ford as fast as we could and came home and got married a few days later, and that was our honeymoon."

At about that same moment, Carroll heard the pilot say they were making the final approach into Nashville and he wanted to thank everyone for flying with them and hoped they all had a great rest of the day. Peggy spit out her gum and wrapped it up in the foil packaging. Trixie pulled out her eyelash curler from her black purse and began to curl her eyelashes. She looked over at Carroll, squinting, and said, "I want to look my best for E.R. He's picking us up."

"Where's Troy?" Carroll asked, assuming he had boarded the plane when they had and was sitting in another area.

"Oh, that Troy," Peggy said. "He got up about five o'clock this morning and jumped in his pickup truck and started driving himself back to Middle Tennessee. That boy will drive any automobile that is handy just as fast as you please, but he is scared to death of airplanes. He says if God had intended for people to fly, He would have given us wings," and she grinned broadly, with a love that comes from years of acceptance of another person's quirks.

As the plane touched down in Nashville and Trixie and Peggy gathered together their belongings, Carroll told them, "I think you're just about the most interesting seatmates I've ever had."

"Can we keep in touch with you, Dr. Carroll?" they asked. She gave them her business card, as she frequently did to those in her audiences, fully expecting never to hear from them again.

"Honey, we didn't know you spelled your name C-a-r-r-o-l-l. That's so cute," gushed Trixie. "I always wanted my name to be Samantha or Rory but Rainey said nobody in East Tennessee where I was raised would have a highfalutin' name like that, so I'd better just stick with Trixie. So I did. "

"The name suits you well," Carroll said as she extended her hand for a farewell shake. "I hope E.R. is there when you get your baggage, and Troy makes it home safely. ' Bye now."

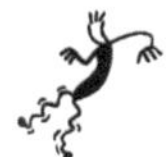

Carroll needed to use the restroom after all the fluid she had consumed on the flight, but she was wary of stepping off the plane, so she opted to use the onboard facility. The plane had almost emptied its passengers in Nashville, and she looked around for another seat, hoping she might get to relax for the next four hours. Luckily, only a handful of new passengers boarded, and Carroll had a row all to herself.

Flying on to LAX, she began to put Trixie and Peggy out of her mind in the same way she did those anonymous voices she encountered in her media appearances. She had sometimes thought it odd she could have such personal conversations with complete strangers one minute and the next minute couldn't have picked them out of a lineup. While her clients and the audience guests believed she was the most compassionate of listeners when they were in her presence, they would have been shocked to know how easy it was for her to compartmentalize them as soon as they had parted company.

After the plane reached its cruising altitude, the captain announced that he anticipated a very smooth flight, so he was turning off the seat belt sign so passengers could move around a little. Stretching out across the three seats, Carroll soon fell soundly asleep, dreaming of wedding cake and pregnancies and dancing. She was glad to be leaving Nashville behind again.

Dancing!

Carroll was startled awake by a clenching in her gut. Her head pounded and her eyes were matted with tears. Shaking her head to try to clear her thoughts and reaching over to retrieve the bottle of Evian she had carried aboard, she fought back the memory.

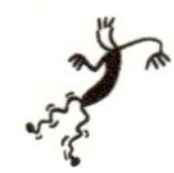

PART THREE: GOD and DANCING

August 1993

Southern California

"Dr. Carroll, I need to ask you something personal," said Barbara, Carroll's long-time office manager, as Carroll stood by her desk in the outer office on Tuesday morning.

Carroll and Barbara were about the same age. They had met when Carroll was finishing her doctorate degree and Barbara was working as an administrative assistant to the dean of the graduate school. Barbara was impressed by the way Carroll was unfailingly polite and friendly to all the women who worked in the university office, in direct contrast to her experience with some of the other women academics who came through that area. When Carroll announced her intention of going into private practice someday, Barbara asked to be remembered if she ever needed someone to run her new office.

Carroll hired Barbara before she knew whether she could even pay her own salary, not to mention that of an office administrator, and she had never regretted her decision. Barbara in turn was one of Carroll's greatest fans, but despite their professional closeness the two women rarely shared personal confidences or socialized together.

"Carroll Murphy is one of the most buttoned-up people I have ever known. I do all of her scheduling, type her final manuscripts, and make her travel plans but even with that I know almost nothing about her private life, and what I do know is only what she has let slip out in a weak moment," Barbara would tell her husband, Sam, from time to time. "But that doesn't matter one iota to me. She would have to beat me off with a stick before I would quit working for her."

Carroll reached over with her forefinger and thumb, clipping a fading blossom from the fresh arrangement in the vase on Barbara's desk. She handed the spent flower to Barbara, whose expectant hand signaled her familiarity with this housekeeping ritual. Since the first week their office was open, Carroll had had fresh flowers delivered to Barbara each Monday, and every day Carroll surveyed the blooms to make sure they were thriving. Early on Barbara had remarked to Carroll that she could do the office gardening herself if Carroll needed to do something else, but Carroll had told her that this was her one effort to take care of something growing and she'd like to do it.

"What would you like to know, Barbara?" Carroll asked, a note of caution in her voice.

"Well, as I think I've mentioned, Cassidy's getting married August 22. It's a Sunday and they plan to have their wedding right after the worship service at our church is over. That way most of the guests she would've invited will be there already, and at the same time we can save a little money by not needing to do any special decorations for the sanctuary. You know, our budget is a little tight right now, what with Sam's being laid off."

She smiled and stuck her chin out just a little.

"Cassidy and Stephen are paying for most everything themselves, but we're doing what we can to help those children out," Barbara added.

"Remind me how old Cassidy is now, Barbara," Carroll said.

"She's twenty-nine this month. I was just out of high school when I had her, but luckily I'd already married her daddy by then and he'll be walking his baby girl down the aisle." Barbara beamed with pride.

"And you wanted to know...." Carroll asked again.

Barbara ducked her head and smiled shyly, then continued. "Well, we're thrilled that you're coming to her wedding and all, especially since I know that every year you take that week in August off, but, uh, I don't really know much about your personal life, and I just wondered if you might be bringing a date with you to the service. You know, so we can have a place for him at the luncheon we're giving afterwards. I mean, you don't have to tell me, but if you are, then we can have his name on the place card next to yours."

Carroll laughed and answered, "Thanks for asking, Barbara. I wish I could say yes to bringing a date, but you know how crazy my life is. I almost never know from day to day where I'll be or what time I'll be home, so that's no way to have a boyfriend. I'll be there but I'll be alone. I know it'll be a special time for your family and I'm glad you've included me."

Carroll pulled out a tissue from the box sitting on Barbara's desk and blotted her nose, then locked her moistening eyes with those of her assistant for a moment before Barbara looked away.

"Guess you'd better have some of these for me at the church in case I start leaking around the edges," Carroll told Barbara who smiled up at her.

"For sure—you and me both," Barbara answered.

"Gotta get a start on the day now," Carroll said, picking up her schedule of clients, and then she made her way to her own office further down the hallway. She could feel Barbara's eyes on her back. *Some things don't need to be explained*, she told herself as she closed her office door.

"Dammit, why does it have to be on August 22—August 22 of all days on the calendar?" she mouthed as her eyes brimmed.

She blotted them with the tissue and drew a deep breath.

"If there is a God, please let me get through that day in one piece," she pleaded, looking out through the east-facing window where the early morning sun was just beginning to shine.

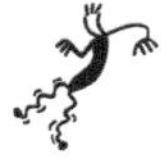

Spring 1994

Carroll usually attended the annual meetings of both professional organizations to which she belonged, but this year she decided to opt out of one of those conferences in favor of attending a different kind of meeting. The modest flyer might not have made the short journey from her mailbox to her desk before being trashed but something about this particular brochure caught her eye, with its colorful family-tree illustration on the front of the tri-fold.

GENOGRAMS DESCRIBE THE PAST—CAN PREDICT THE FUTURE ran the heading. LEARN TO DIAGRAM YOUR CLIENT'S LIFE STORY AND YOU CAN HELP THEM TO MAKE CHANGES.

She picked up her calendar and noted with surprise she was not already committed on the weekend this meeting would take place. Glancing through the program, she saw this would be more of a hands-on workshop, where the participants would be expected to develop and illustrate their own family-of-origin genogram, rather than the more didactic presentation common to other workshops she attended.

Well, that won't be hard for me, she thought, *since I don't have any family. However, it should help me with my clients if I can understand a little more about how family history and culture affects the present interactions.*

She sent off her registration form and put it out of her mind until she arrived at the workshop meeting site in Tucson, one of her favorite locales in the western United States. The Sonoran desert was in full bloom that April. The locals all said that this was the best year in more than twenty for seeing the desert wildflowers because it had been an unusually wet winter for southern Arizona. Carroll put on her walking shoes and headed out through the giant Saguaro cacti. She had been a committed walker for years, meeting her walking partner, Estelle, for three and five mile jaunts in city parks whenever possible, but returning to the desert, especially among all this riot of color, was a special gift for her. In the desert she could walk without encountering the obstructions of city or forest walking trails, and she felt especially serene in that setting.

She requested a single room at the retreat center where the workshop was being held. Having a roommate was always more complicated, and she did not relish the idea of another therapist attendee wanting to stay up all night to process something that had come up during the course of the workshop.

In the opening session, the participants were asked to describe what they most wanted to get out of their time there, both professionally and personally. One attendee said he wanted further insight into his recurring nightmares of family times, and another said she wanted inner peace. Carroll told the group she wanted to understand better the backgrounds of her clients and had no personal agenda, but she certainly supported the efforts of the rest of the group to understand their family dramas more completely.

"Remember, your genogram is a depiction of your family-of-origin—the family you were born into or that reared you, not the family where you live now," instructed the course leader. "It will always be a work in progress because as long as we're still breathing we have opportunities to learn new information and draw new insight from our genograms. So please put today's date next to your family name when you do your genogram, class.

"And it's only necessary to go back three generations—yours, your parents, and their parents—for this workshop. Those are the people who reared you and whom you probably knew and experienced in a personal way. Males are squares, females are circles. In a corner of the genogram write your family rules of conduct—the spoken ones and the unspoken ones," the leader enthused as she dismissed the participants, a scroll of newsprint and a package of marking pens in each of their hands.

"Oh, and one more thing," the leader reminded her pupils, as they started out the door. "How you were named should also be shown. Sometimes we learn a lot about someone's job or role in the family from the name they were given."

Carroll watched as several of the participants paired off, heading to an outdoor picnic table or to one of several groups of chairs set up in clusters near the artificial waterfall in the courtyard. Even though she loved being outdoors, she chose to remain inside and use the dining room, where she could be alone to do her work. She placed her newsprint and pens on a long table and looked around. The tables for eight were arranged in several rows, cafeteria style.

Reminds me of my days at Camp Hopkins, she thought, smiling with the warmth of remembering this happy time in her childhood.

She walked into the kitchen to pour herself a cup of coffee. Opening the refrigerator to look for half and half, she was pleased to see the real product—*not some imitation creamer,* she thought, then she poured enough rich white liquid in her cup to turn the coffee a true mocha, enjoying one of her few splurges from healthy eating. Returning to the dining room, coffee in hand, she stared at the empty newsprint, then picked up a black pen in her left hand and wrote Murphy Family in the top left corner of the paper, then added April 9, 1994 in the upper right corner.

Sipping her coffee, she sat and stared out the window, seeing the animation of some of her fellow attendees who were working in groups in the shade of the trees. She sat the mug down next to the pens and drew a lone circle on the page then took a long swallow of coffee and added a short vertical line that touched the top of the circle and extended upwards. Across the tip of the vertical line, she drew a horizontal line about six inches long, and at each end of this line she drew another vertical line going further up the page. On the tip of the left vertical line she drew a square and on the tip of the right line she placed a circle. She wrote her full name—Carroll Ann Murphy—under the bottom circle; her father's name—Arthur McDonald Murphy—under the square; and her mother's name—Frances Mary Burns—under the other circle. She added the birth years for all three people and a death year for her father, and then put a large X through her father's square, signifying his demise. In her mother's circle she placed a question mark.

Sitting back she thought about the family rules, and then wrote, "Keep your eyes straight ahead so you'll know where you're going" and "We have to be strong for each other." She had just drawn a descending line from her own circle and a horizontal line connecting with it and extending left and upwards when the aroma of frying onions and tomato sauce coming from the kitchen hijacked her brain. *Nobody could make spaghetti sauce better than Brian*, she thought, burying her face in her arms on the table.

By the time the other participants were returning to the meeting hall, Carroll had corralled her emotions and reapplied her game face. Returning from the dining room she noticed most of them were still talking earnestly as they filed into the meeting room, and she watched from afar as they taped their colorful genograms up on the wall. Carroll quietly taped hers at the farthest point in the installation and began to move towards the chairs for the next lecture.

"Not much family, huh?" she heard one classmate ask, and she smiled at him, shaking her head, and then she swallowed hard. She knew her response was not entirely true, but in her head, she heard her father say, "Don't look back." She zipped herself up and sat down.

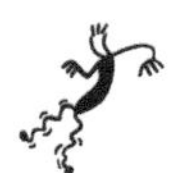

May 1994

Southern California

"Hi, Dr. S.," Carroll said, extending her hand to receive a cup of herbal tea from her mentor and supervisor. "Sorry I'm running late."

She had begun these weekly visits to the home office of Dr. Morris Sutton about five years ago, after meeting him at a regional conference for sex therapists. After he addressed the attendees on "Spiritual Guidance in Sex Therapy," Carroll approached him and asked if he were taking new supervisees. Smiling, he answered, "For you, Carroll Murphy, the answer is yes."

Their rapport was instant, with Carroll proving to be as much the inquisitive student now as she had been in her teens and twenties. Morris Sutton was nearing the end of his pioneering career as a clergyman and sex therapist, a role he had relished but which had also left him somewhat marginalized among his fellow clergy, some of whom found his views on homosexuality and reconciliation to be somewhat more enlightened than theirs. Morris had enjoyed his reformist role in the church until a group of his more conservative pastoral brethren had exercised church politics to strip him of some of his power.

Without knowing much more of his background than this piece, which was common knowledge in the therapy community, Carroll sensed a compatriot and was thrilled to be taken on as a supervisee by him. It was a relationship that proved to be beneficial to both parties.

Carroll brought to each session a case or two that she was treating and for which she needed guidance or she just wanted to bounce around an idea for enhancing the treatment interventions she was using. Most of the time, they also allowed a little time near the end of the supervisory hour to discuss anything in a more personal way. Dr. Sutton was experienced enough to draw a boundary between supervision and psychotherapy, but sometimes they both realized the supervisory process bumped very closely into the therapy process.

"Tell me about the workshop," Dr. S. urged.

"It was good," Carroll answered, "in a weird sort of way."

"Weird? How?" he queried.

"Well, some of the people who were there got really wrapped up in exploring their families-of-origin as the source of their ongoing angst, and a few seemed to have huge breakthroughs in self-awareness. I thought it was all interesting to observe, but...." she trailed off.

"Let me guess. It really had no personal relevance for you, huh, Carroll?"

"Right. You know I have no family left, and what I do remember about my family growing up is all behind me now, so while I could on some level relate to their stories, I just couldn't get into it like they did."

"I see," he said, chewing on the ever present pipe stem he held between his teeth.

"But there was one fascinating piece that did hit home for me."

"What was that?"

"The instructor told us to pay attention to how we were named and what significance that name may have played in our role in life. That part got me thinking. I remember my dad telling me how proud he was that I was named Carroll after his mother. Sometimes he would tease me and call me Carrie—that's what his mother was called—just to see me get angry. Even as a little girl I could not stand to be nicknamed and he knew it would get a rise out of me. He said I'd inherited her fiery red hair and temperament—and her left-handedness. I wish I'd been able to know more about her and about him."

A tear slid over her lower lids and she reached for a tissue to catch it, then smiled at Dr. S.

"We've been talking around but not about your family for several years now, Carroll, and while I imagine you will disagree with me, here's what I think is the truth."

He paused and tried to make eye contact with Carroll but she kept her lids downcast.

"I think you lost your childhood when your dad died."

"Yes, maybe," she snuffled. "But he always taught me never to look back, and my mother taught me to be strong for everyone, so that's what I've done."

Dr. S. smiled and nodded.

"Indeed. I will certainly give them credit for teaching you well. You are an expert at following those rules," he said, as Carroll began to gather her belongings.

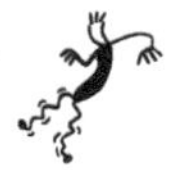

August 1995

Southern California

Barbara was working late, trying to get insurance forms and other paperwork filed.

"I think this is probably the last office in California that still does such things by hand," she had told Carroll and Jeanine during their annual office meeting a few months earlier, "but I'll get us computerized before too long,"

Carroll did not really care how such things got done, as long as she did not have to do them herself, but Jeanine was pushing for computers,

"I think we need to get that new Windows operating system," Jeanine told them. "Despite all the buzz about Apple, from what I can tell Microsoft is about to take over as the new gold standard. Or at least that's what I hear from my geek buddies."

The three new personal computers for the office were soon installed. However, Barbara had not quite come to trust that the data she entered one day would still be there the next, so in the meantime she still hand entered each client transaction in the old-fashioned ledger and filed it in the locked storage closet before she went home each day. She was just completing the last entry from today's clients when the phone rang on Carroll's private line. Barbara answered and parked the call, ringing Carroll in her office.

"Dr. Carroll, I know you're trying to hustle out but I think you need to take this call. It's Ms. Ensworth and she sounds pretty excited."

Barbara put the call through and heard Carroll say, "Hey, Margie, what's up?" before she walked around from her desk and closed the door.

"Carroll Murphy, sit yourself down. You are going to award me agent of the year status. Did I get the book deal of all time for you from the guys at Grondale and Associates! Meet me in a half hour at Batson's and I'll buy you a drink. We are going to celebrate, my dear."

As Carroll grabbed her purse and jacket, she remembered a conversation she had had at Batson's with Margie earlier in the year. Margie was initially resistant to Carroll's proposal to do a book about Lady Godiva, saying the subject was trite and Carroll ought to continue writing the sort of self-help books that her readers had become accustomed to buying. And which, she added, already had made both women a respectable income.

She grew more interested as Carroll explained her plan to do more than historically recount the oft-told tale of Leofric, Earl of Mercia, threatening to raise the taxes on the villagers until his wife, Lady Godiva, told him she would ride naked through the streets if he would withhold the extra levy.

"It's more a book about the politics of female exposure and male compliance than just about Lady Godiva riding naked. You see, Leofric did not believe she would do it. Calling her bluff he agreed to his wife's bargain, and then, quite unusually so for men of medieval times, he upheld his end of the agreement after her now-famous market day ride. She was a powerful woman using whatever means she had to win her position, not unlike what sometimes happens with women today."

She looked at Margie, who was nodding while making a few notes, and then she continued. "This lady is my kind of woman. Smart, tenacious, and a feminist before there was ever a word for such beliefs. Of course, the dutiful husband wasn't counting on Tom, the village tailor, to be looking through a hole in a drawn-together shutter and then going blind after he saw the nude rider. That's the twist that makes the tale a kind of morality play."

"It's a good thing they didn't have personal injury lawyers on every corner back in the 11th century," Margie responded, with a wink at Carroll, who smiled back.

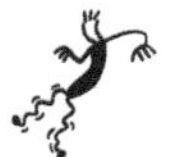

Entering Batson's, Carroll easily found Margie seated in the choice booth in Carroll's favorite neighborhood eatery. She saw that Margie had already started on her first glass of Pinot.

"Tell me," Carroll encouraged, sliding into the booth and facing Margie.

"Darling, it took me ten tries and almost a year of haggling before I got one of those shirts to nibble, but here's a deal I think you'll adore," Margie enthused. "For a while they just did not seem to get it that all the world would want to read a scholarly book about voyeurism and exhibitionism. Then I happened to hit it just right. The wife of the acquisitions editor is a fan of yours on Oprah, and when she saw her husband had brought along your book proposal when they were going to their place in Connecticut for the weekend, she told him to sign you at any cost. Seems he'd never heard of you but she convinced him that all the women in America knew your name and were clamoring to hear more from you."

Margie stuck her nose deeply into her wine glass and savored the bouquet, uttering a satisfied "ummm" before swallowing the liquid.

"Great follow through," she told Carroll, smiling and tipping her glass forward.

Carroll ordered a glass of the house white wine and waited for Margie to go on.

"So, they want the book by last week, and they've given you a hefty advance for your efforts. You look this over and if it's okay with you, we'll both sign on then I want you to use part of the money to go to Coventry and walk the streets and breathe the air of Lady Godiva."

Carroll signed the next day, and when the check for the $50,000 advance arrived a few days afterward, she endorsed it and asked Barbara to deposit it in her research account, adding "And, I hate to ask this, but could you please see what you can do about rearranging my schedule in late October? I'd like to try to get to England for about a week then?"

Barbara smiled and waggled her head a little, knowing how booked with client appointments Dr. Carroll's schedule always was and remembering the guest lectures that had also been squeezed in to her already tight agenda.

"I'll work it out some way," Barbara told her, and Carroll knew she would do so.

"Dr. Carroll is about to become even more famous and more in demand," she reported to Sam that evening. "But I wish she would slow down some. She is going to burn herself out at this pace."

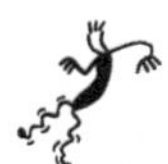

The schedule was altered and the trip was booked for the end of the third week in October. Margie stopped by unannounced at Carroll's office a few days before the journey and asked Barbara to give Carroll the beautifully gift-wrapped present she carried with her—a leather-bound notebook and a box of fine-tipped writing pens.

"Here's to her—to our—success, and to a soon-to-be best-seller," Margie told Barbara. "And please encourage her to have a little fun along with her work. She'll be having her birthday while she's there, and I worry that she keeps her nose too close to the grindstone."

Barbara smiled and shook her head. "That will be the day, Ms. E. That will really be the day when Dr. Carroll Relentless cuts loose and has some fun just for the sake of fun."

The two women looked at each other knowingly and both nodded, thinking their private thoughts about the woman they both admired.

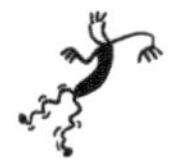

Early October 1995

Southern California

"Won't be here in two weeks, Dr. S." Carroll told her mentor at the end of their session as he was reaching for his appointment book. "I'm off to the mother country to investigate peeping toms."

"Carroll, you are heading for burnout if you keep up this frenetic pace—clients in your office one hour, lecturing to graduate students the next, hopping a plane to Chicago the next, traveling abroad to research some topic for a new book or paper, working out in the gym or taking a yoga class the next. I'm exhausted just trying to mentally keep up with your schedule."

She gave him a rueful smile and responded, "Yes, I realize I'm at risk, but I have to keep dancing." *Strange I would use that word—dancing*—she thought, *since I don't plan to ever dance again in my entire life.*

She handed him her empty tea cup and hurried out of the office.

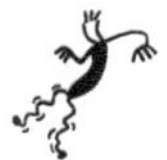

Late October 1995

England

Carroll had been in Coventry for a week, determined as always to make the very best use of her time by staying on task, and she had succeeded in finishing her research a few hours ahead of schedule. This newest book, tentatively entitled *The Naked Truth about Lady Godiva*, had been the most enjoyable one she had done, and the visit to this quaint English town had allowed her to put together in actuality some of the pieces she had previously only been able to view in her imagination. The excitement she felt was both welcome and a little unfamiliar.

Her bags were packed and stowed, waiting for the cab ride to the train station. Her shoulder bag that doubled as a purse was bulging with notes she had taken and in her hand, she held Margie's gift, the leather-covered notebook.

Maybe I'll nip into the pub and write a few sentences. Margie's sure to ask me if I took time for self-reflection in the midst of my research.

She turned the idea over in her mind, and then decided to forego introspection for now. *I'll have time on the train for writing,* she thought, tucking the notebook next to the papers inside her purse. *I'd better say goodbye to the lady now.*

For almost every minute of her time in this Midlands city, Carroll had kept her head burrowed in archival material. The research librarians had been enormously helpful, giving her access to ancient documents and regaling her with tales of modern-day Godiva-wannabes when she would take a break from her scholarly tasks. It was clear to her that the residents of Coventry felt especially gifted to be the center of this centuries-old legend, and she was pleased to share their enthusiasm for a good story.

Pausing for one last look at the Lady Godiva statue standing in the center of Coventry, she looked up at the rain-clotted sky and ran her fingers through her perpetually frizzled hair, finally deciding to give it a twist on the top of her head with the hair scrunchie she retrieved from her purse. *I have almost two hours before I have to catch the train back to London, so maybe I'll have a look around the inside of the cathedral.*

As was her usual practice Carroll was traveling alone, intent on making her own decisions and keeping herself company. Whether it was for research, speaking engagements, or vacations, she was invariably a lone traveler. "And I like it that way," she would tell her colleagues who always shook their heads at her declarations of independence.

Let them think what they wish. For me, the best thing is to go it alone, Carroll told herself.

Since arriving the previous Monday, Carroll had felt conflicted about playing tourist. She had spent some of her research time in the library at Coventry University, whose grounds adjoined those of the St. Michael's church and cathedral at Priory Street. While she had walked around the perimeter of the old cathedral's shell as part of her self-orientation to Lady Godiva's habitat, she had not set foot inside the building. *I'm here on someone else's dollar and I need to stay on task*, she'd told herself when she was tempted to venture into the bombed-out ruins that remained after the Germans strafed the area in November 1940. *Besides, I think religion is the reason for most of the problems of the world, and I refuse to pay homage to another religious relic or to see another old rugged cross.*

Something kept urging her to walk on up the steps to St. Michael's main entrance, but something else held her back. Inside her head, she heard her yoga instructor telling the class, "Lean into your resistance," and she smiled. *Once a certain person embeds herself in your mind, they are there forever.*

"These are called introjects," Carroll would tell the students at the university where she lectured. "It is the job of people who care about you, like a parent, to insert themselves in your mind so when they're not around they can still give you advice. Sometimes that works for you and sometimes it works against you," she would add, and the students would usually chuckle in recognition of their own personal introjects.

Turning for a last glance at the Godiva statue, she crossed Priory Street slowly, heading for the university, then she took a deep breath, pivoted, and climbed the two tiers of steps leading to the main entrance of St. Michaels. After buying a ticket and field guide from the volunteer manning the sale booth, she walked across the porch that joined the new church with the old one and then she stepped up the few steps into the bombed out remains of the old cathedral. Carroll looked up though the roofless opening and smiled to see the late afternoon sun breaking through the dark clouds, flooding the floor of the almost empty shell with shadowy images. She turned left and walked slowly along the remnants of the Cathedral wall's, observing the relics, old and new, that stood in sparse appointment in what she imagined had once been a magnificent building. She paused briefly at the Altar of

Reconciliation, reading that the day after the bombing, the then-warden of the church had seen the cross-like figure of two charred roof beams that had fallen and were lying in the ruins. The warden recovered it, she read, as a symbol of hope and resurrection, themes which subsequently had become the heart of the Cathedral's ministry

She turned from the altar area heading toward the Bell Tower at the other end. Somehow it had withstood the Luftwaffe destruction. Completing the rectangle she rounded the interior corner and walked along the west wall. Approaching the corner through which she had entered, she gasped. Standing directly in front of her was a bronze statue displayed about waist-high on a brick pedestal bearing an identifying plaque. Nearby was an empty stone bench and at the base of the statue were several small wreaths made of artificial flowers placed in no particular arrangement. She stood staring at the statue, unmoving in the pool of sunlight at its base, then recovering from her momentary paralysis, she stepped back and placed her hand over her mouth. Shivering despite the sun's warmth, she drew her jacket tightly around her, and then with caution she again stepped closer to the statue.

Two solitary bronze figures, a man and a woman, about life-size, each kneeling on bended knees, embraced each other, the man with his right arm encircling the woman's waist while the left one pulled her head onto his shoulder. The woman's arms held the man around his shoulders, forming a bridge between them. Their faces were downturned and unseen as they leaned into each other. Carroll focused her gaze on the arched space under their connecting arm bridge, feeling completely drawn into the opening.

"They've crossed a space and given in to something," Carroll heard herself whisper. She reached out and stroked the shoulder of the female figure. Even though the statue itself was made of bronze, there was softness to it. *Great symbolism, hard and soft merging.*

Moving closer to the statue she read the identifying plaque.

"Reconciliation," she mouthed.

The wording, in English on one end of the plaque and Japanese on the other, described the gift of the statue to the cathedral as a token of reconciliation to commemorate the fiftieth anniversary of the end of the Second World War. An identical statue had been placed in the Peace Garden in Hiroshima by the people of Coventry, she read.

"Josefina de Vasconcellos. A woman sculptor. Who knew?" Carroll remarked aloud.

"Yes, love, one of the most famous sculptors in the world. Ninety years old she is and still working—did the original of this piece when she was a mere 73. Lives a stone's throw from here," said the middle-aged man who was standing next to Carroll. He picked up the Leica dangling from a leather strap around his neck and snapped a couple of photos.

"Just been here a little more than a month, this statue," he continued, never looking directly at Carroll or seeming to expect an answer from her.

"I like to come here in the afternoon and shoot when there's Jesus light coming in—too many shadows from the tower there in the morning."

Then tipping his cap in Carroll's direction, he moved on around to the other side of the statue, snapping away.

"I usually throw out 99 of 100 of the lot when I print 'em, but ah, it's jolly good when it all comes together. Good day, love."

Carroll watched him move on down the nave towards the bombed out altar then she stood back from the statue again taking in the image in her mind. She felt her heart leap in her chest and she covered it with her hand, patting it gently. For once, she wished she had broken her own rule about traveling lightly and had brought a camera herself. *Even one of those throwaway jobs would be good here.*

"I'll see if I can buy a postcard at the station before I leave," she told herself.

Later, seated on the train, she pulled out the color postcard and stared at it. She felt slightly light-headed and fearing she might faint, she bent down to reach her purse, now stowed under her seat. She quickly placed the card inside a zippered pocket in the bag, glancing briefly at the leather-covered notebook that beckoned to her from the depths of the purse before again dismissing the idea of self-reflective writing.

"That was an odd feeling," she muttered, then she closed her eyes and dozed, awakening as the train pulled into King's Cross station. She hailed a cab outside and within the hour, she was in her hotel near Heathrow. Boarding the plane back to Los Angeles the next morning, she put the statue out of her mind and slept soundly for most of the long flight home.

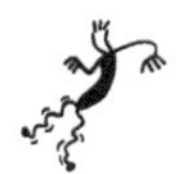

March 24, 1996

Diary entry

Dearest Carroll,

Today would have been your dad's seventy-second birthday. I wonder what he would have thought of the way things are in the world today if he had lived.

I always said I'd never seen a better looking, more pathetic soldier than Art was on the day I met him. He'd been evacuated from France and by the time he arrived in my hospital unit, he was severely dehydrated and in shock from the blood loss. I could usually predict who would make it and who wouldn't, and looking at Art, I fully expected him to leave under a sheet. His pluckiness surprised everyone in the unit, and before long he was throwing himself off the bed and into the makeshift wheelchair someone had rigged out of an old wheelbarrow. His stump wound healed slowly and soon he was telling jokes to the other soldiers, and generally forcing everyone to do a better job of getting well. "Can't go back and do it over—just gotta keep moving on," he would say.

You are my precious beloved child.

Love always,

Mother

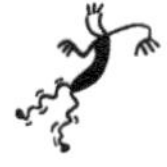

Monday, August 10, 1998

Southern California

"I don't care if it does cost $10 a pill," gloated Mike, a bearded, slightly pudgy lawyer in his mid-fifties, whose balding pate confirmed to Carroll's eyes that the male hormone had been strongly at work in this man.

"To get a hard-on I can trust again is like being reborn! I'd go without food before I'd go without that little blue baby."

"Then what's happening in your life that you need my help with, Mike?" Carroll asked.

"Well, I just can't seem to get my wife to want to have sex with me as often as I want to with her," he answered, fidgeting in the comfortable tweed club chair opposite Carroll. He paused and picked at a tuft of thread on the arm of the chair that worried his thumb and index finger, twisting it until he gave up the struggle to break it off.

"Does she know you're now using Viagra™?"

"I don't think so. I figure it's none of her business. Now I've wasted about $50 taking pills those times when I thought I might get lucky, and then something would happen and she'd go to bed early or pick a fight with me or some such thing. There I'd be with the flagpole run up, if you know what I mean, and no flag to hang on it."

Carroll grinned and consulted her mental notes on regional idioms, wondering if Mike had been raised in the Midwest. In graduate school she had found it fascinating that euphemisms describing sexual material often could be used to pinpoint the geographic locale of the speaker's family-of-origin. She mentally catalogued this phrase for follow-up later on.

"So, you've not told your wife about your use of an erection aid medicine, and she's not cooperating with your schedule of seeking sex with her? Is that right?"

"Well, when you put it that way, it is right. But I just didn't want her to know I'd been struggling a little with my manhood, and I thought once I showed up with things working well again, she'd be impressed."

"I can see how, from your point of view, your solution would seem to make sense, but I wonder, Mike, if your wife may have figured out what you're doing and she's resenting that you've kept her in the dark. And when she's feeling resentful or angry, then she withdraws sexually from you."

"Is that what's happening, Dr. Carroll? I'd never really thought she might want to know."

"Well, I talk to a lot of women who tell me what they most want from their relationship is to be truly a part of what's going on. Since taking Viagra™ means a man has from one to four hours to use the erection it brings on, it seems to me your wife needs to know so you two can plan when intimacy will take place. I call this true oral sex—using your mouths to communicate about sex rather than letting your genitals do the talking. As we age, Mike, our bodies don't react sexually in the same ways they did when they were younger. So it's very important for couples to communicate with each other and plan for sexual encounters rather than waiting for their bodies to rise to the occasion."

Carroll was momentarily surprised by what she had just heard herself say. She always prided herself on using the correct anatomical terms in her client sessions, and her last four words did not fit that standard. She felt a slight blush starting in her chest and working its way up to the mid-point of her cheeks. Quickly regaining her composure, Carroll allowed the beginning of a smile to light on her mouth, and then she reframed the interaction.

"Does it make sense to you that your wife may be feeling left out?"

"Yes, and I'm willing to tell her, now that you've mentioned it to me. If things are no better, then I'll suggest she come in here with me and maybe you can help us talk it over. Thanks."

"Okay, Mike. See you next time."

As the office door closed, Carroll turned and glanced out the window behind her. The setting sun passed behind a cloud, turning the western sky a brilliant quilt of pink, gold, green, red, and yellow, and Carroll turned her attention to the next client on her schedule and to all she needed to get done before her flight to DC on Wednesday.

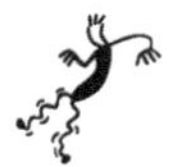

Monday, August 17, 1998

Southern California

Thank the Universe, I'm finally home, Carroll thought, exhaling slowly.

Washington and Nashville seemed to be on another planet by the time she opened the door to her small condo in Pasadena. Her message light was blinking, and she fielded the calls as she sorted through her mail.

She slept fitfully but got up on the first beep of her alarm clock and showered and dressed.

I'll have to let the hair just dry on the go. Doesn't matter what I do, it always looks the same anyway.

Her coffee was brewed and ready by the time she reached her kitchen, and she reached into the refrigerator for half and half, mixing it in a commuter cup, before heading for her car.

I'll grab a muffin and maybe I can make it by nine. I'm going to need all the caffeine I can get the next twenty-four hours. Why do I schedule myself so tightly?

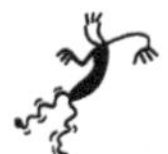

"Dr. S., I really need your help. You would not believe what happened to me on the plane yesterday."

Dr. Sutton had been encouraging Carroll to give up her coffee habit, so he always had herbal tea ready for her. Sitting down with the replacement cup in her hands, she began to fill him in on her recent encounter.

"I had another one of those nightmares, but I'm almost used to them by now. The thing that's really getting me, though, is there were these two women on the Nashville segment, and they pinned me in my window seat and talked nonstop for more than two hours."

"What bothers you the most about that, Carroll?" he asked.

"The fact that I actually almost liked those women! Never in my life have I voluntarily spent time with people like that. And besides, you know how I despise Southerners, especially the Nashville version."

"And these were Sonny's kin?"

"Almost," Carroll answered, grinning.

"Well, caught as you were in that seat, you weren't exactly volunteering for the duty, Carroll. Let's look at this a little deeper, shall we?"

Dr. Sutton reached for his pipe and began to chew on the end. He had given up the use of tobacco after his heart bypass surgery a few years earlier, but he still loved the feel of holding the bowl in his hand and having the tip of the pipe just between his front teeth.

Carroll smiled at the view from her seat. With his pipe floating over the cascade of his white beard and his round belly protruding from his lap, her clinical supervisor reminded her of a little statue of a gnome that had been in her favorite aunt's yard when she was a child.

"As we've discussed, Carroll, one of the greatest risks of therapy is the mismanagement of transference. You know, the way you handle the people who push your buttons. The ones who make you act out of character for yourself. Now, I know these seatmates were not actually your clients, but in some ways you seem to have become hooked by their stories," he started.

"Yes, you and I have been over this ground lots of times in reviewing my work with clients," Carroll sighed. "The whole time I was pinned in by them, you were right there in my head, asking me why I couldn't just let go of the bait."

Carroll stretched out her long legs and took another sip of her tea.

"So, what was your answer to what I was asking in your head?"

"I didn't have an answer! That's why I was so befuddled. Usually I can rely on reading my magazines or just keeping my silence or—as in Sonny's case—the perfect stare and one-liner to get someone to leave me alone, but they didn't seem to catch any of the cues I gave them."

"Maybe you weren't actually signaling them very strongly," Dr. S. said, smiling, as he tapped the empty pipe bowl in an ashtray on his desk.

Carroll took off her glasses and rubbed her eyes. She didn't want to look at this issue much deeper at the moment, since she had a full caseload of clients to see in the office and then had to prepare for the redeye flight to Chicago.

How will I find time to get to the gym today, too? she wondered.

"Why don't you try writing about this in your journal, Carroll? I know you're not much on keeping this kind of diary, but you might discover more about this with some self-reflection."

"I'll try, Dr. S. I'll try."

She knew she probably wouldn't try, but she did not want to disappoint her mentor. She just did not like writing about herself. When Jeanine had proposed that they and a couple other therapists meet at lunch once a week to talk about their progress in *The Artists' Way*, Carroll had gamely joined up, but after doing a few chapters, she dropped out of the group.

"I don't like doing those morning pages. I guess I'm just a failure at journal writing," she told them.

In her head she heard *Don't look back.*

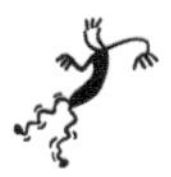

Tuesday, August 18, 1998

Live from Chicago

"Ladies and gentlemen, please welcome Dr. Carroll Murphy, better known to the women of America as The Sex Lady!" Several women in the audience let out a whoop, and Oprah turned and gave them her trademark stare.

Carroll entered the stage waving confidently, wearing her signature navy gabardine slacks and a cornflower-blue cashmere twin set, with a strand of pearls at her neck and two pearl studs in her ear lobes. Her hair flowed unfettered and her porcelain skin, with just a trace of freckles across her nose, glowed under the heavy lights. No one seeing her on TV would have guessed she was approaching her fifty-second birthday. Her on-camera vibrancy always amazed her clients and friends who experienced her as quiet and even a little reserved in their presence.

"Dr. Carroll is going to help us understand why our president is in so much hot water with Congress, not to mention hanging in the doghouse with Buddy while Hillary decides whether to ever give either one of them any more table bones," the show's hostess said.

The audience roared as the monitors around the studio flashed the now-familiar picture of the forty-second president being nuzzled by Buddy, his chocolate Lab, while Hillary glared through clenched teeth at the two of them.

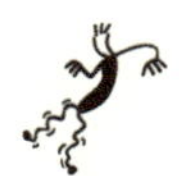

Wednesday, August 19, 1998

Nashville

"Peggy, you won't believe this. Honey, it's her. It's *Dr. Carroll.* She's on *Oprah* today. Well, I mean I guess she was actually on it yesterday, but, oh well, you know what I mean. Oh, God, she didn't even tell us that was where she was going. I sure wish I had asked her for her autograph."

Trixie was frothing into Peggy's answering machine.

"Honey, call me just as soon as you step foot in the door and get those boys of yours fed. Oh, hurry, hurry, hurry. I can't wait!"

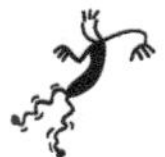

Peggy almost never got to watch *Oprah* when it aired on Channel 4, since her workday did not end until after the show was over, but she taped it nearly every day, along with her favorite soap, so she could watch both of them before bedtime. Listening to Trixie's message as soon as she got home, she heated Troy's plate of leftover meatloaf and mashed potatoes and green beans in the microwave and told him she would eat later.

Troy was flipping through the channels on the television, hoping to get some news about the goings-on in Memphis the previous couple of days, without any success. He always promised himself he would be at Graceland some year on August seventeenth, but the time had not yet come for him.

"I swear, that is the most disgusting sight a body ever saw," he cursed aloud to the images of the president recanting his previous denial of his affair with *that woman,* while Hillary and the Gores stood painfully behind him. "Slick Willie is nothing but a no-good ass-chaser, and we all ought to be ashamed to have such a creep in the White House!"

He turned on the VCR and began searching for his collection of Columbo reruns. Even though he had seen every one about fifteen times, he still leaned forward with anticipation when Columbo was closing in on the suspect. "Now there is one smart dude," was always Troy's admiring description of the ever-sly detective.

Troy Jr., who usually got home from football practice a few minutes after his mother got home from work, shared his dad's enthusiasm for effective police work, and he would nod along in cadence with Troy. Peggy would sometimes stand to the side of them, marveling at the remarkable way genetic characteristics were passed down.

She and Troy and Lisa Marie moved to Nashville in the late 70's in pursuit of a better life than that promised them in East Tennessee. As Troy's mechanical skills became more sought out, he opened his own shop. After the unexpected birth of young Troy following a thirteen-year dry spell, the family moved from their small tract house into their three-bedroom dream home in Camelot Downs.

Peggy started college when Troy Jr. was in first grade, determined to get her bachelor's degree in nursing. It took her almost ten years to complete, working full-time in the clinic, but at her graduation Troy, Lisa Marie, and Troy Jr. were enthusiastic supporters in the audience as she moved toward the podium to accept her sheepskin.

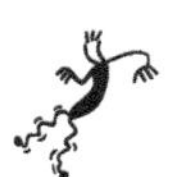

Peggy settled herself on her bed and put the VHS cassette in the tape player, and then she phoned Trixie so they could discuss their two favorite celebrities in person. Over the years, the cousins had been coordinating their viewing of Oprah on tape so they could discuss it scene by scene, and by now they had this ritual down to a science.

"Oh, sweetie, isn't she something?" gushed Peggy when she heard the tape begin to cycle. "Just think, it hasn't been hardly forty-eight hours since we were on that plane right next to her, and now there she is in the flesh right up there in the Windy City with Oprah. Oh, I wish we could call her up and say hi, but I guess it's pretty much out of the question since they taped this show yesterday."

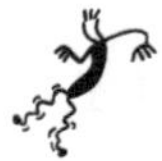

"So, why has our president gotten himself in such hot water, Dr. Carroll?" asked Oprah.

"Well, it's difficult to know from afar—and please remember, no one from the White House has consulted me—but there is a lot about his behavior that seems pretty typical of the men and women I treat for the disorder called sexual addiction."

"Do you mean to tell us this leader of the free world is sitting up there in Washington acting like a teenager with raging hormones because he has an addiction to sex?" Oprah faced the camera and mouthed *I don't think so*. Her audience applauded and nodded in agreement.

"I know it seems pretty impossible to believe, but just for a moment let's look at his behaviors and compare them to what we currently know about sex addiction. First of all, before anyone in the professional audience out there jumps on me, I am aware there is not officially in the DSM any diagnosis called 'sex addiction,'" Carroll said.

"So, let me get this right. You are saying the president has a diagnosis which does not exist, and that explains why he is in such trouble? In Nashville, where I grew up, they had a name I can't say on television for guys like this." Oprah gazed at the audience, who clapped furiously.

Carroll waited for the audience buzz to quiet. Her media training had emphasized the importance of the guest setting the agenda by only saying the two or three things that had been rehearsed, no matter what question the host might ask. She knew she needed to get back to the topic in the next thirty seconds or she would lose her opportunity.

"Oprah, I know you and your audience are very familiar with eating disorders."

The television hostess hesitated, nodding.

"Well, just in the same way some people can severely overeat or can starve themselves, some folks can act sexually in extreme ways, with serious consequences."

"Like being in a lot of trouble with the Congress or with their wives?"

The audience laughed.

"Yes, but the important thing to be aware of is just having a lapse of judgment does not amount to addictive sex. There has to be a pattern over a long period of time. Usually, we also see attempts to stop the behavior, which may work for a while, but then the pattern starts over again, usually ratcheting up to more risk with each new occurrence."

"Well, from what we are hearing, the president didn't just start acting this way once he got in the White House."

The studio camera zoomed in on a woman in the audience who was nodding emphatically.

"Yes, that's what I mean about a pattern. Also, there are a number of factors that might set someone up for this particular disorder."

"Like what?"

"Usually there are genetic factors in someone's background. Another addict, especially a parent. A history of emotional, physical, or sexual abuse, or sometimes a deep loss that occurred at a critical period. A sense of poor self-esteem, although that may be covered up with certain personality types."

"A narcissist, for instance?"

"Could be, since a narcissist is almost incapable of taking responsibility for himself, blaming others for almost everything."

"Okay, folks, there you have it. Do you think our president is a sex addict, or just another wayward husband who got caught? We have to break away, but when we come back, we'll take calls and see what the studio audience thinks about all this."

In the studio, the mostly-female audience began to chatter to each other, clearly having their own opinions about the reasons the White House was in such uproar. Two women seated next to each other had tears brimming in their eyes.

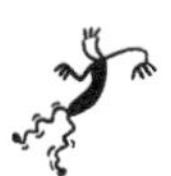

Peggy pushed the fast-forward button, barely noticing the flying images of toothpaste and cleaning products zooming across the screen.

"Tell me when you're ready," she instructed her cousin.

Trixie moved the phone to her other shoulder, holding it tightly with her chin, while she dabbed polish on her chipped nails.

"Sex addiction? How does a guy get off with that so-called diagnosis?" Trixie pouted, almost dropping the phone as she reached for an orange stick.

"Excuse me, sweetie, but I think getting off is what landed him in this stew, so to speak." And they both howled into the phones.

"Honey, I don't know what Oprah's friends called it when she lived here, but where I live, we call it being a sinning philanderer. I am about an expert on the subject, after being married to Joe and Frank. Now there were two losers if there ever was one. Those boys could not keep their flies zipped up if an even halfway attractive female came within sniffing distance. Do you remember what that Frank did after me and E.R. moved in together? He would call up and act like he didn't know it was me on the phone, and then he would suggest all sorts of lewd things he would like to do to me. Finally, one day when he called, I had about had it, and I said to him, 'Thanks for applying for that position, but it is already filled. Don't call back.' And he slammed down the phone and never did call back."

Peggy responded, "Well, I don't know for sure, but I think I have heard of that diagnosis. Awhile back, one of the doctors in the clinic got in bad trouble with the hospital for fooling around with a couple of techs after hours. And before long, we heard through the grapevine he had been shipped off to rehab somewhere in Texas. He came back a really changed man and actually apologized to us for all his misbehaviors. I would never have believed it if I hadn't seen it with my own eyes."

"Lord, honey, those doctors will do anything to save their rich asses."

"Well, maybe so. I don't know," Peggy answered.

"Ready," Trixie said, and they pushed the play buttons on each of their remotes.

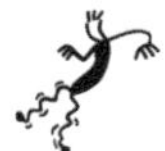

"So let's see what our callers say about this so-called diagnosis of sex addiction. Jolene from Waukegan, hello. What do you think about this topic?"

"I think he's a liar and he's going to hell for all this trashy behavior and making the United States the laughingstock of the world."

"Well, thanks, Jolene. There's no doubt whose side you are on."

As the camera panned the audience, a few women grinned and clapped, but others just registered their confusion or shock.

"Robin, from Gary, Indiana. Hello. Do you think our president is a sex addict?"

"I don't know. But when I was a little girl, I had an uncle who couldn't keep his hands to himself, and later on, I found out he did this to all the girls in the family. I think he must have been really sick to have done what he did."

"Dr. Carroll," Oprah asked, "are sex offenders and sex addicts the same thing?"

"I'm glad this question came up, and I'm so sorry you had to go through those experiences, Robin. Some sex addicts are sex offenders, but most are not."

The cameras caught the image of an attractive thirty-something woman in the audience leaning into her companion's ear and rapidly speaking. The friend was nodding and laughing.

"Let's see what our audience has to say."

Zooming in on one of the women who earlier had been in tears, the camera began to record, "I'm the wife of a sex addict. My husband was a minister, and I thought he was the most unlikely person to ever have a problem with sex. Then I learned he had been involved with several women in the congregation whom he'd been counseling. That was five years ago, and our family has been to hell and back, but we're both in recovery now and I think we'll make it."

The hush in the audience was perceptible.

Carroll thanked the woman for sharing her story, and then she continued. "Certain professions seem to be more vulnerable to this disorder than others are. In my practice I see clergy, lawyers, physicians, and especially entertainers, since I'm in Los Angeles."

"Well, I bet we could all guess who some of the latter are," chuckled Oprah.

"We have to break, but when we come back, Dr. Carroll will tell us what can be done about sex addiction."

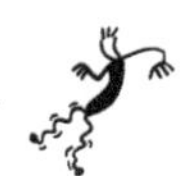

Trixie's chin firmly clamped the phone in place, while she spread her fingers in front of her chest, turning them first to the right then to the left to check for misses in the mid-week nail repair job.

"Honey, if you ask me—and I know you didn't—what can be done about those scum is you can cut off their balls. I was too scared of Joe to consider doing anything like that, but Frank is just lucky he still has a deep voice. I thought about it again last weekend, after what he said to me at the wedding. Imagine, someone with two college degrees being that gross."

Peggy was tethered to the twenty-five-foot phone cord attached to the wall behind her bedside table. From there she could walk around the bed, picking up Troy's discarded work pants and shirt and carrying them to the laundry basket in the closet.

Why didn't I train these boys to pick up after themselves? she asked herself for about the hundredth time, sighing loudly. She remembered the empty toilet paper rolls and the *Playboy* magazine she had retrieved from under her son's bed when she last cleaned there. From her vantage point, it seemed hard to tell the difference between a teenager in heat and the actions of a sex addict.

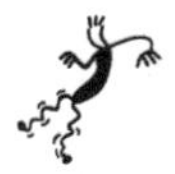

August 20, 1998

Nashville

By Thursday morning, every person who worked with Trixie had heard about her famous new friend.

"You met a real-life sex therapist? Oh boy, I bet you learned some new tricks from her!" gushed Vicki, who worked at the reception desk next to Trixie at the Beautique Salon and Day Spa.

"Well, no, honey, she didn't say much along those lines. She seemed a little uptight really, but I guess she just keeps her guard up. A person like that probably has to be mighty careful about who she talks to and what she says. She gave us her card, though." Trixie dug into her purse, searching for the errant business card.

"See!" Trixie held the card aloft and adjusted her reading glasses on her nose so she could better focus.

"Carroll Murphy—Carroll with two R's and two L's, if you please." Trixie ever so slightly tilted her nose and quaffed a tiny sniff of upper crust air before continuing.

"Carroll Murphy, PhD, Certified Sex Therapist, FAAST—I wonder what those letters stand for?—blah-blah. Los Angeles, California; e-mail, drcarroll@thesexladyonline.com."

"She gave you her e-mail address?" squealed Vicki, as some of the salon customers waiting to be called looked aghast.

"Oh boy, do I wish we had e-mail here. We're lucky we even have computers for handling payments, much less Internet service in this salon. Maybe in a couple of years," pondered Vicki.

Continuing, Vicki urged, "Let's write her a letter at her office and ask a question, Trix. This is the chance of a lifetime."

By then, a couple of the stylists had also joined in the excitement and echoed their curiosity.

"Boy, will my honey be impressed if I tell him I got the word directly from the Sex Lady," cooed petite Carla. "Sometimes he watches her on Oprah when he is home in the afternoons, and he tells me how cool she is."

Calvin poked his head around the corner from his station in the main salon. Seeing his mother, he gave her a big hug. His almost-six-foot frame, broad shoulders, and dark wavy brown hair momentarily blotted his mother from Carla's view.

Carla could tell he had already been working on his own hairstyle, from the freshly gelled crest he had fashioned.

"How's my Trixie?" he asked his mother.

"Honey, when are you ever going to call me Mama like your brothers do?" pouted Trixie.

"Well, you don't look old enough to be anybody's mama, beautiful, and I have never called you anything but Trixie in my entire life, so why would I stop now? You look lovely today. What's this I hear about you meeting the fabulous Dr. Carroll? She is way cool."

Calvin's handsome features caught the attention of both women and men in the Beautique Salon, and he was careful to flirt equally with both genders. His tight jeans, always neatly pressed with a crease, topped by a fitted shirt with the neck unbuttoned enough to reveal a handsome mane of chest hair, served him well in keeping a full clientele. It didn't hurt that he was also enormously talented, and every customer left his chair feeling like royalty. Often the women would comment to Trixie as they were leaving, "I sure would like to marry that son of yours."

"So, are you going to write her a letter, Trixie?" he teased. "I can think of some things *I* would like to ask her."

"Now, hush, Calvin. You are making your mother blush, and that is not good for somebody who gets those hot flashes." It was hard to tell whether the glow on Trixie at the moment was from an estrogen surge or that of a proud parent. But she was tomato-red from her mid-chest to her crown.

"Ooh, I know what I am going to ask her," purred Nadine, whose slicked-back raven hair and high heels were legendary in the salon. "I want to know how I can get Ron to slow down and wait until I'm ready before he gets off."

Trixie looked around, hoping she still had a job. Turning to face the waiting-room chairs, she glimpsed only the hemline of a pair of Armani slacks escaping into the spa.

"Well, la-te-dah, honey. I guess *they* don't ever have any sex problems like the rest of us mortals do," quipped Trixie, and all the girls howled.

"You tell 'em, Trixie," Calvin cooed, as he pecked his mother's cheek before heading back to his station.

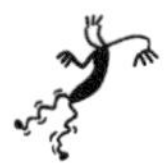

When Trixie arrived with the completed letter the next morning, the entire staff at Beautique gathered for the reading.

Dear Dr. Carroll:

All my friends at the salon are so excited I met you on the plane. They want me to ask you some questions. Honey, I hope this will be all right with you. After all, I guess you get asked questions all the time, since that is what you do for a living. And we know you are really smart because we see you all the time on Oprah, and you always know exactly what to say. Well, here goes, honey.

Number one—is there a way to make a guy last longer? Nadine says her guy bought some of that stuff you—well I don't mean you personally—I mean a guy rubs on his thing and it's supposed to deaden the sensations. She said it didn't seem to make much difference, and then she just kind of got deadened too.

Number two—is it true a girl can come more than one time—I mean, during one time of doing it, can she get off more than one time?

I hope you will write me back.

Your friend,

Trixie

With her fans gathered round, Trixie glowed and raised her scepter.

"Oh, Lord, honey. My hands were just shaking when I wrote that. I mean, I never have ever written a letter to a famous person before. I mean, unless you would consider the letter I wrote to Elvis back in 1977, and then he died before it even got there. It came back to me with some handwriting on it. 'Return to sender.' Oh, mercy, did I ever cry about that."

Carla and Nadine hugged Trixie and told her how proud they were of her for writing such a nice letter.

"Well, to tell you the truth, I was up half the night redoing it on that old electric typewriter we have at E.R.'s place. I decided to use French script because I thought it would be more personal that way. I am sure glad Miss Higgins showed us how to do that on a typewriter, but I wish I had one of these word processors at home."

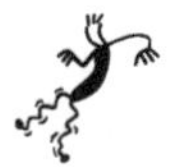

September 8, 1998
Southern California

As usual, Carroll arrived at Dr. Sutton's office a couple of minutes late, her coffee mug in hand and her hair on end. She swallowed hard from her own cup, then accepted the proffered tea from her mentor, seating herself and removing her papers from the briefcase.

"Dr. S., I think I'm in trouble. They wrote me a letter."

"A letter? What did it say?"

"Well, actually it was a really appropriate letter, considering the source. Trixie—she's the Dolly Parton look-alike—wrote it. I'm guessing Peggy or somebody else helped her get it together, because I can't imagine she could type or spell that well."

"So what do you think you'll do, Carroll?"

Dr. Sutton leaned back in his desk chair and looked over the half glasses on his nose. He really enjoyed seeing his favorite therapist try to work things out for herself under his guidance.

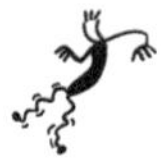

September 15, 1998

Nashville

The salon was closed as usual on Sunday and Monday, but as soon as the back door was unlocked on Tuesday, Trixie burst in, grinning from ear to ear and waving in front of her an unopened rectangular white envelope, bearing a Los Angeles postmark.

She grabbed a cup of coffee in the break room, then picked up three packets of sweetener and began tearing them open. Carla looked on in amazement as Trixie dumped the ingredients of one yellow, one pink, and one blue packet into her cup. Trixie took a long drink and licked her lips, then turning to Carla with a wink, she said, "Just trying to be on the safe side, honey, in case I could get cancer from one of them."

Carla frowned, leaning over to untie her running shoes, as she prepared to change into her working ones. "A good glass of carrot juice would be so much better for you, Trix dear," Carla offered, but the only part of Trixie still nearby was the scent of her English Rose cologne. Carla remembered Rainey had been a big fan of English Rose, especially Yardley's, so the girls in the salon had tracked down a supplier of Yardley's and had given Trixie a large bottle for her mother when she was last hospitalized. Trixie was finding she had a fondness for Yardley's, as well.

In the front desk area, a crowd of stylists had gathered. "Oh, lookee here what I have! I know it's been three weeks since I wrote her, but she's written back. It was about all I could do not to tear this open on Saturday when I found it in my mailbox, but no sirree bob, I said to myself, 'Trixie, honey, we wrote that letter all of us together, so it would not be right to open it up and read it until I am at the salon with all those other girls. And boys.'" Trixie surveyed the crowd for Calvin's face, without success. She felt a little relieved because she was not sure she wanted her oldest son to hear her read Dr. Carroll's response.

Within a few minutes, all the stylists and receptionists had surrounded Trixie's desk in the lobby, and she ceremoniously began to slice the top of the envelope, being very careful not to disturb the return address or the postmarked thirty-two-cent stamp.

"Oh, ladies, this is so exciting. But I think I'm about to have one of my hot flashes," said Trixie. She reached in the drawer under her desk, produced a fold-out fan, and began to beat the air around her ferociously. Beads of sweat gathered in her temples, and her neck started to blotch, spreading up to meet the sweat line. She removed the cardigan sweater that covered her matching short-sleeved pullover shell. The large plastic pearls encircling her neck were unceremoniously deposited on the desktop, along with their companion clip-on earrings. Several stylists smiled at each other, noticing how Trixie was beginning to imitate her new celebrity mentor's wardrobe. Trixie's ample chest strained to remain inside the shell as the hot flash passed over.

Carla whispered to Nadine, "If she would stay off coffee, her flashes wouldn't be so bad. Just a little soy in some carrot juice will nip those in the bud."

Dear Trixie:

It was nice to hear from you. I trust both you and Peggy are doing well in Nashville—you at the salon and Peggy at the clinic. Please say hello from me to everyone there.

"Oh, honey, did you hear that? She says hello to us all," Trixie exhaled.

"Hello, Dr. Carroll," the gathered audience echoed.

Things have been a bit hectic here with some travel and speaking engagements, so it took me several days to get to your letter and to reply. Yes, I get asked these types of questions all day long. So here goes.

In response to the first question—"Is there a way to make a guy last longer?" —Nadine's experience is fairly typical.

Most humans, especially guys, want to find a magic cream or pill that will make sex last longer, but in fact there is not yet any such pill or cream. It sounds like what Nadine's guy used was a product which probably contained some numbing substance that also numbs the inside of the vagina, so neither person is getting much of a sensation. And then what usually happens is the guy just goes ahead and climaxes as he always has, but neither he nor his mate feel it so intensely because of the numbing.

Guys, especially young guys, are just doing what nature designed for them to do—get up, get in, get off, and get out before some predator comes along and tries to kill them off. So, in Nadine's case, the couple is really working against nature to try to last longer.

There are ways to do that, though, and most of these ways have been in practice for hundreds or thousands of years by people who live in India and China, for example. We call these practices—

"TONTREAK—no. TAHNTRICK—no—"

Trixie's eyes widened as she stumbled over the word. "TAN-TRICK" a shout from the back of the room corrected her.

"*TANTRICK, tantric sex,*" Trixie continued,

and they involve learning ways to breathe quietly and become more relaxed, as opposed to more tense, during the experience. When that happens, a guy can last longer.

"Well, I never. I mean, who ever heard of relaxing when you're getting excited? I just always held my breath waiting for it to be over," Trixie confessed, waving the fan and sipping from the water glass someone had slipped in front of her.

I hope Nadine and her guy will consider looking into some of these. There are several books available and I have enclosed a reading list if they want to do a little homework on their own.

"Here it is if anybody wants to do some homework," and Trixie waved the pages above her head.

From the back of the assembled group, Vicki shouted, "Take that list to your book club next month, Trix. Bet those ladies would like to review one of those titles!"

Trixie fanned herself harder.

"To tell you the truth, I'm about worn out with reading all this advice. And I sure do wish she would use plain old English, but I guess if a person has as many initials after their name as she does, they just can't help themselves from using big words. Carla, honey, would you come up here and read the second answer?"

"Sure. Hand me the letter," said Carla, coming forward.

> Now to question number two—'Is it true a girl can come more than one time in the same sexual experience?' Yes, that is true, but it doesn't always happen, even to the same woman who is with the same partner and doing the same thing. We are just beginning to learn how complex a woman's sexual response system is. Women have thousands of nerve endings—lots more than men have in the penis—which allow women to enjoy a wide range of sexual gratifications.

"Hey, hey, let's hear it for female superiority," said Carla, raising her fist in a power salute.

> Most women tell me they are content sometimes to just 'be' in the encounter, whether or not they ever reach climax. When men hear this fact, they are usually amazed and sometimes unbelieving, because to a guy the goal of a sexual encounter is usually to climax—so to look at the female point of view is difficult for most men.

Carla fixed her gaze on Rudy, the only straight guy who worked in the salon.

He retreated a little, shaking his head. "Not this guy. I'm forced to hear a woman's viewpoint about every hour working here. That one she can't lay on me!"

> A guy is pretty limited to one or sometimes two climaxes per event, but a woman can actually have lots of orgasms, depending on her wishes for that to happen and how relaxed and at the same time how stimulated she is.
>
> Hope this helps.
>
> Yours truly,
>
> Carroll Murphy, PhD, CST, FAAST

"Oh, my goodness," breathed Trixie, fanning herself and mopping sweat from her temples with a towel someone brought her from the shampoo area. "Maybe I will give up coffee after all, Carla. I guess I'd better be getting to work. Anyway, she did answer our questions. Next time I'm going to be a little more private, though. I sure am glad Calvin wasn't here to hear it all."

The front lobby erupted in applause. "Way to go, Trixie!"

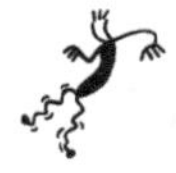

October 29, 1998

Diary entry

Dearest Carroll,

Even when you were very small, you were always such a different kind of child—using grownup words and reading far beyond your years. And so fiercely independent! Guess you got that from your dad. When your teacher suggested bumping you ahead to second grade, even though you had just turned six, we talked it over and he urged me to let you do it. I always thought he was pushing for you to be both his son and his daughter, so I encouraged you to pursue more feminine activities, like ballet. I admired the ways dancer's legs were so shapely and the way they could move with such grace, but you thought otherwise about ballet. You said you liked the sound of metal taps as they hit the floor and the little swishes they made with a brush step. To your six-year-old mind, ballet was slow and tedious but tap was vigorous and loud. Tap dance it would be.

You are my precious beloved child.

Love always,

Mother

P.S. I have your copy of The Little Engine That Could, which you got for your seventh birthday forty-five years ago today. I found it a few years ago when I was clearing things out for my move. You must have read that book hundreds of times when you were little. I'll keep it for you in Grandfather Burns' old trunk, just in case you decide to come home again.

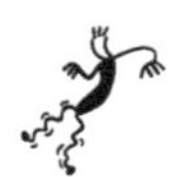

November 1998

Southern California

Dr. Sutton was well into his seventies and beginning reluctantly to slow down from his once vigorous life. He had bounced back from his bypass surgery four years ago and had resumed his regular tennis matches and his gardening, so he had been surprised to learn his blood pressure was out of control at his last doctor's visit. He was having a hard time adjusting to the new medicine he had been given, and he had had to cancel the standing Monday appointment with Carroll last week. Feeling stronger now, he was eager to renew the relationship with his favorite student.

He handed her a cup of tea and leaned back in his office chair, smiling.

"Did your new friends invite you to go buck dancing with them on your birthday in—where is it they go? Bethel?" he teased.

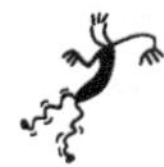

A couple of weeks earlier Carroll had brought in Trixie's second letter for her session with him.

Dear Dr. Carroll:

Thank you so much for answering my letter. Everybody in the salon learned so much from what you said. I read it to Peggy on the phone that night and she said to tell you 'hey' when I wrote back, so here is a 'hey' from her.

I don't really have a sex question for you, but maybe you can help with just a plain old life question.

Now you remember I told you about my living with E.R. and that we are not married or anything. Well, E.R. does not think it is proper for two people who are not married to have sex, and honey, that is just fine with me because I am too old and too worn out to care most of the time.

But, honey, I sure do like to dance. And after all that buck dancing up at Faye's wedding, why I told Peggy after we got back here I was just about determined I would find someplace around here where we could dance, and Lord, honey, wouldn't you just know one of the men by the name Donny Ray what works at Troy's garage sings bass every Saturday night in a bluegrass band, and that band was playing at a local community not too far from where me and E.R. live, so we all decided to just go there and see what we could see.

And, honey, it was sure some good old-time dancing going on there. And we stayed through until they shut the doors at 10:00.

But, honey, here's the thing. That E.R. just would not dance with me because of the name of the place where we were. It was "Bethel" and he said it was against his religion— he was raised Nazarene—to dance in such a holy-sounding place.

Now there was this whole group of folks from the Church of Christ that was there—and their preacher was there, too—and they were not missing even one dance. And they said they all planned to march themselves right into their church the next morning, so I could not for the life of me see what was eating up E.R.

Now, honey, I know you are not a preacher or anything, but with all those initials after your name, maybe you can help me. Do you think there is anything wrong about dancing in Bethel?

Your friend,

Trixie

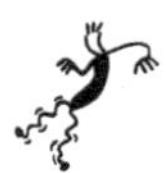

"Did I go dancing? You've got to be kidding. First of all, they're in Tennessee and I'm in California. And even if I were there, you more than anyone know I would never dance and for sure not in public. Why would you even ask me such a thing, Dr. S.?"

He lifted his feet out of the pile of sarcasm puddled under them and answered, "Oh, just hoping you'd tell me about your conflict with dancing and how it plays into this drama with your new friends."

"I don't do friends. You know that about me, too."

"Yes, so you've told me lots of times, but I keep hoping I'll get lucky and find out the real reason."

Carroll drew her breath in and held it for a long moment, and then released it slowly.

"I've had some bad experiences with so-called friends. And I don't like Southerners. They're all a bunch of rednecks. As for these ladies, I'm just curious about some of the ridiculous things they tell me about. They're like unenrolled research subjects for the new book I'm thinking about writing—you know, the one about sexual idioms and euphemisms in North America—and they're also sort of like soap operas for me. The Trollops give me a little comic diversion."

"Okay, I'll buy that for now, but I don't understand why you spend so many hours doing research on all their problems and then send Trixie detailed answers. You don't respond to other letters you get from the public in this way, do you?"

"No, but this is different," she protested.

"How?" Dr. Sutton asked.

"It just is." Carroll's voice was barely audible.

"Tell me about the last time you danced, Carroll," Dr. S. invited.

Carroll blinked hard to stanch the tears. She drew a long breath, holding it for almost thirty seconds before letting it out slowly, letting her abdomen rise and fall with the breath.

Dr. Sutton leaned forward to hear her whispered answer.

"Well, Brian tried to get me to dance when I met him. But I said, 'No dancing. Not now. Not ever.' And after a while, he stopped asking."

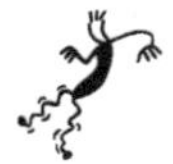

Summer, 1967

Carroll had always had a quick mind and a love of learning, but when she entered the University of Oregon for the fall term in 1964, she attacked her studies with a new vengeance. In one class, she was required to read *Man's Search for Meaning* by Viktor Frankel, which became a particular favorite of hers. She estimated she had read it at least five times by her graduation in 1967, always trying to puzzle how the worst times of one's life can somehow be the most meaningful.

After graduation she went to Hawaii with some of her U.O. friends who lived there. Having spent years waiting tables in college, she knew she could easily get a summer job on Oahu and also have some time to play a little before starting grad school on the mainland in the fall. She and her girlfriends quickly learned they could spend their off time on the beaches of some of the biggest Waikiki hotels by masquerading as hotel guests. Even with their recent feminist indoctrination in Eugene, they were not above using a smile or flirt to get past the desk captains, when needed.

Brian always liked to say he spotted her first, but the truth was she had seen his taut, athletic body with its bronze sheen lying beside the pool sleeping when she first walked out to the lanai. She was curious that he seemed so peaceful, unlike the other thousands of Vietnam veterans who streamed into the islands in search of booze and women after their stretch in the jungles of Southeast Asia. Most of the ones she had encountered in the bars and on the beaches were starved for companionship—and they especially wanted to get laid. Having sex was about the farthest thing from Carroll's mind in the summer of 1967, so she would look them in the eye and icily tell them she was not available.

Brian had awakened with her eyes on him, like a couple of the radar trackers he relied on for guiding his plane back to the carrier. Lifting his head, he shielded his eyes from the late afternoon sun and searched the horizon for the source of the beams he had felt. Her red hair glowed in the low-slung sun as her lean, tall body helped prop up a coconut tree at the edge of the patio.

She was wearing a lime-green polka-dot swimsuit, and her flawless complexion needed no makeup or lipstick in Brian's mind. She turned and started back to the lobby of the hotel, clutching her beach chair and towel in one hand and the ever-present book bag in the other.

He stood up so quickly he almost toppled with dizziness as he hurried to get ahead of her, gallantly swooping in an exaggerated bow to allow her to pass through the door he had just opened. She laughed self-consciously, feeling her pulse quicken as she brushed her hand against his arm. She dropped her sunglasses, and Brian bent to retrieve them for her. Her breath halted and she touched her face and turned her eyes downward, very uncharacteristically, she would later think.

Brian handed her glasses to her. Standing upright again, he seemed to her even taller than she had first thought, and his bright white teeth sparkled as he smiled and spoke for the first time.

“Hello, ma’am. Can I give you a hand with those things?” He reached to help her carry her chair.

“No. Yes. I don’t know,” she mumbled shyly, and he lifted the beach chair deftly through the door. His southern drawl assaulted her ears, but at the same time, she could not stop listening as he softly introduced himself.

“I’m Brian Fogarty, ma’am. Lieutenant J.G., U.S. Navy, at your command,” he said with a snappy salute. His smile just about brought her to her knees, and she felt herself start to moisten between her legs.

“And just what name do you call yourself, if I may be so bold to inquire?” he asked.

“Carroll. I’m Carroll. With two R’s and two L’s. C-A-R-R-O-L-L,” she mumbled.

“Very pleased to meet you, Miss Carroll with two R’s and two L’s,” he teased. In most cases, she would have huffed off at even the slightest teasing, but she couldn’t move and just stood there giggling.

Brian cocked his head back and looked at her. “Now I declare, what’s a pretty little girl like you doing standing in this big old hotel at five o’clock in the afternoon with hardly any clothes on and giggling, again, if I can be so bold, Miss Carroll with two R’s and two L’s?”

Carroll started laughing. She couldn’t remember laughing like this for a long time, and certainly not since she had been an adult. She felt like a fifteen-year-old who had just been smitten with her first crush. She put her hand over her mouth and looked at Brian, and he reached down to cover the swelling in his swim shorts with his towel.

"Now, ma'am, I think we are both feeling the heat of this place, so I believe we better both go to our own rooms and shower and then meet down here in one hour and see if we still like each other."

She and Brian were inseparable for the next five days, and on the day before he was due to return to Vietnam, he took her to Diamond Head at sunset and proposed to her.

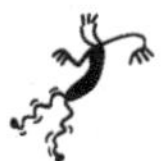

They were married in California in 1968, shortly after he completed his tour in Vietnam. Brian voiced his surprise that Carroll had no family she wanted to invite to the wedding, but Carroll told him her father had died when she was six, and from the time she was a freshman in college she had had nothing to do with her mother. For all she knew, she told Brian, her mother might be dead, which was how she wanted things to stay. The warmth of his big family and all the brothers and sisters who embraced her sometimes took her breath away, but she tried gamely to fit in with them.

Janie, her best friend from childhood, was her only attendant at the service in the little chapel on base.

"I don't know what the Pope will say about this," laughed Brian's sister, Ellen, squeezing Janie's hand just before the service began. "First we have a non-Catholic service, and then we have a Jewish matron of honor."

"I guess we'll just spend our final time in some limbo place," echoed Brian's brother, Ed, hugging the three women.

Carroll wobbled a little at this sudden familiarity. Growing up, she often felt smothered in the same way when she visited Janie's home. "I don't know whether I can take all this hugging from your family, Janie," she'd said then. "Sometimes I think they have to hug someone every time they leave the room to go to the john." The girls laughed, knowing it was almost true. "Just breathe," Janie retorted. "It won't kill you to hug somebody." Carroll wasn't so sure. In her household, hugs were perfunctory and only happened when someone was going away to some distant place.

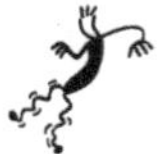

Carroll and Brian moved into a tiny apartment outside La Jolla, close enough to U.C.S.D. for her to commute easily and within range of Miramar, where Brian was instructing pilots at the newly established TOPGUN school. For the first time since he had left the Naval Academy, he could sleep a little later in the morning and come home for dinner. At age twenty-six, life for Brian Fogarty and his new bride was about as sweet as it could get.

Carroll attacked her master's course work as relentlessly as she had her undergraduate studies. Until her marriage, she had always thought she would focus her graduate work on the indigenous people of the Pacific Rim, studying their mating patterns in generally the same way as her role model, Dr. Margaret Mead, but with Brian in her life, she had shifted her focus to social psychology.

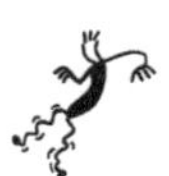

September, 1969

Carroll was typing the final version of her master's thesis when the doorbell of their apartment rang. It was two o'clock in the afternoon, and she sensed immediately something dreadful had happened. Opening the door, she saw the uniform of a Navy chaplain.

The chaplain said, "Ma'am, I regret to inform you Lieutenant Fogarty has been killed in a crash at sea while instructing a student pilot."

Carroll remembered nothing else of that afternoon. Brian's family attempted to encircle her with their love through the three-day Irish wake in his hometown of Birmingham, Alabama, but Carroll sleepwalked through it all. When the Navy honor guard brought her the folded flag from Brian's coffin, Carroll fainted. That night she miscarried the nine-week-old fetus that Brian had never known existed. The Fogarty family insisted the fetus be christened and buried beside Brian. By the time the brief funeral mass was ended and the tiny grave covered with dirt, Carroll had turned the page to a new chapter in her life.

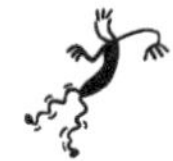

"So, I just work, Dr. S. That is the only thing I trust in life. I work and I keep to myself and I let others do the dancing."

Carroll had hardly moved in her seat as she told this part of her story to Dr. Sutton. As she finished and looked up at him, reaching for the mug of tea he was refilling for her, she absorbed a little of the warmth reflected from his eyes.

"You were deeply wounded by that experience, Carroll. Maybe it's time for you to begin healing."

"I really think I'm over it, Dr. S. It's been almost thirty years now."

She began to gather her papers and put them into her briefcase. "Gotta go—my public is waiting for me."

"OK, see you next week. Oh, by the way, you didn't ask, but in case you ever want to know, Bethel means house of God. I guess E.R.'s Bible leaves out the parts about the Israelites dancing in the house of God."

Carroll grinned and shook her head.

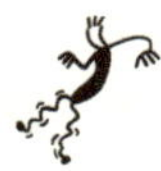

March 1999

Los Angeles

Barbara handed Carroll the schedule listing her clients for the day and watched as Carroll frowned, guessing that she was anticipating her appointment with the Whitehurst couple in the six o'clock slot. She knew her boss's reactions well enough to recognize that this twosome could still be a thorny duo in the usually easy-going routine of their office. Even though things were less rocky today than when they'd started therapy several months ago, both women had learned to expect some fireworks.

Barbara was just shutting down her ledgers when Larry arrived a few minutes early for the visit. He sat in the waiting room flipping the pages of a magazine while waiting for Marjorie, who as usual was about ten minutes late. Barbara buzzed Carroll to let her know they were both now arrived, and then she picked up her purse and left the office just as Carroll came out to greet the couple.

"So how have things been going since your last visit, Marjorie and Larry?" asked Carroll.

"Well, I've tried to follow the suggestions you gave about putting our relationship ahead of my business commitments, but sometimes nothing I do ever seems to be good enough for her," answered Larry.

"I see. Marjorie, what is your view on this?" asked Carroll.

Marjorie was still dressed in her tennis clothes, and she struggled to arrange her short skirt over the tops of her tanned and toned thighs. She was wearing a white tennis sweater casually slung around her shoulders, but now she removed it and slipped her arms into it, straining to pull its front lapels together to insulate against the chill of the air-conditioned office.

"Oh, for about the first twenty-four hours after we were here, he did make a few weak attempts to relate to me, but then it was back to business as usual. So I just quit expecting anything and put all my energy into my tennis game. He doesn't have a clue how lonely I am or why I think the tennis instructor is so cute."

"And have you tried to put in words for him those feelings of being lonely, Marjorie?"

"Yes, but he is just like my father. All he thinks about is making money and if he's not at work, he's on his computer or his cell phone talking to someone about business."

"So you were lonely in your family growing up, Marjorie, just like you feel now?" asked Carroll.

A tear began to slip from Marjorie's carefully made-up left eye, but she hastily blotted it, checking the tissue after each blot to see if her mascara had smeared.

"Larry, did you know that Marjorie was lonely as a child?"

"Well, yes, I guess I did. But it's hard to remember that when she's so busy comparing what we don't have to what her family had. I have worked my fingers to the bone to try to give her the big house and fine furniture and great vacations that she seems to expect, but it's never enough. I even paid for her to get her boobs enlarged and her nose tapered down. And just look what she did to our marriage, carrying on with her tennis teacher, a no-good bum who preys on all those women in their skinny little shorts and their tight shirts. And to top it off, she's stopped having sex with me again. If I have told her once, I have told her a hundred times I don't need anything fancy from her, but a good screw once a week or even a blowjob would help my mood a lot."

"I did not carry on. I met him at Starbucks a couple of times, and we went for a drive along the beach highway in my convertible, but that's as far as it went," wailed Marjorie.

Ignoring her, Carroll turned back to Larry.

"So you feel angry and betrayed, and maybe even misused by Marjorie's displaced affections, is that right, Larry?"

"You damn well better believe I do. And I am not going to take it for much longer!" exploded Larry.

Marjorie's face paled and her dark brown eyes clouded as she absorbed what her husband of twenty years was saying.

"OK, go ahead and sue me for divorce. I will bury you. Once the world hears about your little stash of porn on the Internet and the way you've been carrying on with your secretary, you'll lose that big-time place as the head of the Deacon's Committee at the church, not to mention what your stockholders will say when they find their golden boy is really made of brass."

"Well, this all sounds familiar now doesn't it? Let's sit back for a minute and breathe," said Carroll.

Over the months since this couple had first consulted her, Carroll had taught them to move from the initial outburst to the message the outburst was trying to convey. This was a major struggle for most couples because it was so much easier just to fight with each other than to get at the underlying issue.

"It seems to me that you prefer to blame Marjorie rather than to acknowledge that you're also scared and lonely, Larry," Carroll observed. "In therapy terms, we call that 'acting out' your feelings rather than speaking them."

Carroll stood up and lifted the cover page on the large pad of newsprint sitting on the easel next to her chair. "Let's take a look at your family genogram again, Marjorie and Larry. As you remember, we've been through some of this before, and it's always been helpful to retrace the roots of your relationship so we can all better understand what's going on today."

"Your dad was always at the office or away at some business-related meeting and your mother consoled herself by shopping for new houses. That's what you have told us previously, right, Marjorie?"

Marjorie dabbed at her lower lids and nodded, biting her tongue.

"And then your dad began having an affair with his secretary when you were in high school and you were the one who discovered their secret, when you took his Mercedes out for a joyride and found his girlfriend's wallet in the glove compartment. So you made a vow to yourself never to be in your mother's shoes and then, lo and behold, here you are today. Correct?" asked Carroll.

"Yes, but things are different today. I've not been spending Larry's money on houses and clothes. I hardly ever buy anything for myself, and he's the one who wanted our big house. I was happier when we lived in the smaller one where we started out."

"Tell me about how things were with you and Larry in those earlier years, Marjorie."

Larry leaned over and offered his wife a tissue. Marjorie glared at him and yanked the tissue out of the container, pulling a wad of others out at the same time. As the clot of tissues fell to the floor, Marjorie's hand brushed Larry's, and for a moment their eyes met, then she looked away.

"Well, for one thing, they were calm," began Marjorie. "Never in my life had I experienced anything like peace and quiet in a home. Where I grew up, someone was either yelling at someone else or running in or out of the room. It was like Grand Central Station."

"So the home you and Larry established felt safer than the one where you grew up?"

Pausing to reflect, Marjorie slowly answered, "I guess so. I didn't know whether my parents would stay married another day. And then one day, they really did explode, and from then on it was all-out war. Of course, they would never really get divorced because that would not have been socially acceptable, but they might as well have. In fact, from my point of view, I sometimes wished they had divorced instead of just putting all of us kids through purgatory."

"Go back to what you were saying about the differences you and Larry set up in your lives," prompted Carroll.

"Yes, one of the things that attracted me to Larry was his calmness. He never got rattled, and he never once yelled at me while we were dating. We promised each other we would never go to sleep angry at each other, and until the last year we never did."

Shifting the newsprint pad slightly to highlight his part of the genogram, Carroll noted, "Larry, you've already told us that your parents had a long, happy marriage and as a child you never heard them disagree or saw them work out any differences."

"Yes, I guess I thought that was how all families behaved. Looking back on it, they must have had some times they weren't in total agreement, but as far as I knew then, all was peaches and cream."

"So what did your parents' relationship teach you about working out problems, especially in light of what you and Marjorie are going through?"

"I guess it didn't teach me much of anything, except to expect there wouldn't be any problems," reflected Larry.

"And what did Marjorie's upbringing teach her about working things out?"

"That there should be lots of drama and blaming and huffing around, especially behind the façade of the house."

"OK, now I want you to tell that to Marjorie. And I want you both to follow the ground rules we've already established. No name calling. No storming out. No interrupting until the other person is finished. Agreed?"

"Agreed."

"Agreed."

"Marjorie, when you blame and threaten me like you did earlier, I feel really hurt and bewildered. I see that you are repeating a pattern that you learned growing up, and I feel just like I did in my own family as a kid when I could never be perfect enough. I really don't have a better way of dealing with this, since my folks never taught us how to work things out, but they also didn't teach us to explode like yours did. So, a few minutes ago when I exploded and blamed you, I felt I'd become your dad and you'd become your mother. Does that make sense to you?"

"Yes, Larry, that makes a lot of sense to me. I can't stand it when I see the two of us becoming like my folks. I really want us to be like your folks—or rather like I used to think your folks were."

She smiled and shot a sideways wink to Larry. "I know Dr. Carroll is sitting over there saying, 'Marjorie's family is conflict-prone and Larry's family is conflict-avoidant,' so I'll say it for her since we've been paying her big bucks to teach us these things."

Both of them giggled and looked at Carroll, who was nodding and smiling.

"I'm sorry that I pulled out the porn stuff from my gunny sack. That was dirty pool. The same thing's true about my not wanting sex. I do use that tactic when I feel lonely and want to get even with you."

"Thanks, Marjorie, for your amends. Part of me knows that you're speaking from your hurt when you threaten me, but another part of me fears you'll actually do something rash. I can see how my actions trigger that part of your background."

A tear fell from Marjorie's now-very-mussed lower eyelid and she did nothing to stop it. Both Larry and Carroll sat back and allowed her the space to cry.

Looking at the genogram, Carroll noted to herself that one of the strongest family messages that had been instilled in Marjorie was *You must never show your deep feelings*. She felt a shiver up her spine and shifted in her chair until the feeling subsided, then she continued. "Today, Marjorie, you have someone in your life who cares about you and who had some of the same dynamics in his growing-up years as you had, so he can truly empathize with you, even though it takes a little guidance still to help him—and you—get below the surface pain that you both have. Is that right?"

"Yes, that's right. And I would so much rather be able to feel my feelings than to have to stuff them inside. Looking back, I think I grew up in a den of insanity."

"Well, in lots of ways, my family was just as insane. We may not have been down and dirty like yours, but we certainly weren't truly resolving things either. And I also want to change things in our family in ways that my and your parents could not do," Larry offered.

Carroll enjoyed those moments when her clients could stand back from their own situations and see the bigger picture.

"We all have genograms," she would often say. "Even if we're not conscious of them, they're directing our lives."

The vaguest of tremors climbed back up her vertebrae, but as she had learned to do so many times, she resisted it.

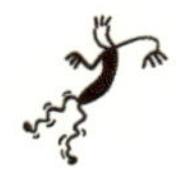

PART FOUR: REDEMPTION and DANCING

January 18, 2000

Park City, Utah

Carroll preferred to take solo vacations, so she would have the option of connecting—or not connecting—with anyone she might meet along the way. She'd heard lots of stories about single women so desperate for companionship that they made bad decisions in their search for a mate, and she didn't want any cumbersome entanglements in her hectic life.

She was an expert at making small talk when necessary, but usually she would dine alone and be asleep in her own bed by ten-thirty. She always brought her professional papers and journals along with her on ski vacations, since she never knew when she might get stranded by a blizzard and would need to fill the time in some useful way.

She relished being one of the first on the lift in the mornings, because there was nothing more freeing than making new tracks on a brilliant winter morning in the Wasatch. She skied in Colorado through the seventies, when Americans were just discovering the sport and immediately loved that she could ski all day in almost complete anonymity, ski suits and sunglasses effectively hiding one's identity, which suited her desire to keep her personal life pigeonholed. Then in 1982, a client remarked about a new resort that had just opened outside Park City, Utah, and she decided to investigate it.

From her first trip, she was captivated. She could rent a condo in Deer Valley near slopes that offered enough of a challenge to keep her entranced all day. By the late 1980's she'd had enough professional success that she could afford a somewhat more luxurious ski experience—not like the bare-bones resorts where she'd learned to ski.

"Are you single?" she heard a male voice ask.

"Yes, and you?" she replied.

"Works for me," the skier grinned.

Carroll smiled, recalling her naiveté a few years ago when she was asked the same question and, thinking the skier was coming on to her, she had huffed off. Only later did she realize his question simply had to do with lift seat availability.

As the ski lift swung slowly around, each of them crouched to receive its seat under their buttocks. Carroll kept her gaze fixed on the seat cushion while her hand gripped the side bar. She had learned in an early ski lesson some years back that the secret to getting on and off the ski lift easily was not to get preoccupied with distractions that might cause a ski to get crossed or a pole to catch in the snow.

Her companion glanced to his right and Carroll could feel his eyes on the auburn tresses cascading over the collar of her turquoise ski jacket. One of his ski poles caught the edge of snow just in front of the STAND HERE sign, and the pole tipped forward out of his reach.

Both of them looked over their shoulders at the now-receding pole as they were swept forward towards the crest of the mountain. Turning his head back, her seatmate sighed. "Oh, well, I never much liked that pole anyway."

Carroll's muffled giggle wafted to his ears across the frozen valley, which was speeding away from them. He reached to lower the hand-and-foot bar. She removed her leather ski mittens, carefully attaching the tether hooks to her ski parka. Keeping her silver mitten liners on over her chilling fingers, she reached inside her ski pack to retrieve a tube of Chapstick, which she generously smoothed over her drying lips.

"Thanks," she said. "I usually don't need the bar down, but I will defer to you, since you are the handicapped one of us."

Carroll replaced the mittens on her hands, beating her palms together to restart her warming circulation. She pulled her neck gator up slightly around her mouth and readjusted her ski cap against the north wind that shot across her face as the ski lift began to ascend the ravine. Exhaling, her breath fogged her goggles momentarily, but just as quickly they cleared, giving her a clear view of the valley below through the orange lenses.

"Mitch is the name," he said, extending his hand to Carroll.

She shook it but remained silent.

"Are you going to poke fun at me all day?" Mitch asked.

"All day? You must be smoking something. I don't expect you can keep up with me for even one run," Carroll shot back, sending him a sideways glance. She liked the fact he was not wearing goggles and she could see his eyes, and the raccoon print around them confirmed to her he was a regular on the slopes.

"Where're you from?" he asked.

"California. And you?'

"Oh, I have a little cabin up here in these hills."

Carroll had heard that line before. It always seemed to her when a man in this town wanted to impress a woman, he would refer to his home as a little cabin, when in reality the home might have thirteen bedrooms, a live-in butler, and a shooting range in the basement. She'd concluded it was a guy thing, and she entered this phrase into her burgeoning mental catalogue of idioms.

The quiet of the snowscape was pierced intermittently by the grinding of the lift cable as the upward train passed the empty downward one. Below them, Carroll traced the tracks of a rabbit from just inside a stand of barren aspens to the other side of the still-groomed Solid Muldoon run. It would be after lunch before that run would emerge from the shadows, but it was a good run in the afternoon when the sun was shining on its slopes.

The lift began to descend to its point of exit and Mitch asked, "Ready?" then lifted the foot-and-hand rest so they could dismount.

"Guess I'll need to make a quick run down the hill for my pole. Catch you later!" He saluted as he tipped his sunglasses down over his eyes and pointed his skis downhill, sending up a spray of powdery snow onto Carroll's ski pants.

"In your dreams," Carroll mouthed into the incoming breeze.

Her experience had shown that most men she met on lifts were determined to show off their skill—or lack thereof—and she had no interest in any competition. Either that or they wanted to have sex.

Not my type, she thought. *Definitely not my type.*

She watched him disappear over the crest of Solid Muldoon and then poled over to the downhill run connecting to Silver Lake Lodge. The memory of her recent seatmate had evaporated by the time she was seated on the upward bound Sterling Lift and the runs of Bald Mountain where she intended to spend the rest of the day.

Putting her skis in overnight storage at 4:00 that afternoon, she glanced over her shoulder and saw Mitch skiing in for the day also. She watched as he removed his skis and hoisted them and his poles onto his shoulder and headed in her direction, making his way to the parking lot. She knew he hadn't seen her. Just as she reached the stairs leading down to the locker room they came face to face. He nodded but said nothing.

He's pissed, but he'll get over it.

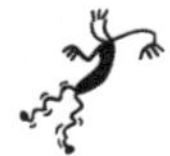

January 19, 2000

It wasn't as though Trixie had never tried to use the Internet before, but up to this point she had only used the computer at the beauty salon receptionist desk to do her online business. This had worked out pretty well in the beginning, since the only person she regularly corresponded with was Peggy, who also could occasionally use the computer at work to send a brief response to Trixie's email.

For Christmas the month before Calvin had given his mother a personal computer for her home use. Trixie had been more surprised by that gift than any other she had ever received.

"Lord, honey, you would have thought I was going to have a conniption when I opened up that card under the tree and it told me there was a cow in the garage. I mean, why in the world would I want a cow? But I could see by the glint in Calvin's eye it wasn't exactly the kind of a cow you'd see out in the pasture. And I sure was glad of that! But, honey, I for sure was not expecting to find a brand-new computer sitting inside a big old box with Jersey spots on it. I don't know how in the whole wide world people come up with some of the stuff they do, but Calvin just told me not to worry about it. It was the packaging the company had always used, and it helped them stand out from the crowd. And I guess he's right about that," she reported to Peggy in their nightly phone check in.

Peggy was glad no one had given her a computer. She didn't really like using the ones at work, and she couldn't imagine she would ever want to have one in her own home. She felt the same way about cell phones. Watching her coworkers pull their phones out of their purses as soon as they clocked out, she thought, *Why would I want to get in my car and immediately start up a phone conversation with someone, especially after I have been talking to people all day?*

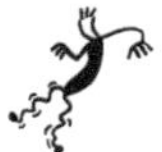

Calvin helped set up his mother's new toy on a small wooden desk he was recycling. E.R. did not think Trixie had any business getting a computer when she knew hardly anything about them, but by the time it was completely installed, he gave up the argument.

"Honey, I never thought I would use those 96 words a minute I learned to type back in Miss Higgins's office-skills class in tenth grade, but it sure has stuck with me. I can type faster than I can think, and I just never know what's going to come out when my fingers start to fly," she confided to Peggy.

Trixie couldn't believe how much there was to do out in cyberspace—it was as if the boundaries of her narrow Tennessee world had been completely blown away. Sometimes she would find herself chatting with people all over the world.

"Peggy, honey, I'm beginning to wonder if there are any sane people in outer space. Last night, I was talking to three people at once in a chat room, and the next thing you know, one of them—who I thought up until then was just the nicest man in the world—he turns out to be the Creep of the Year. Do you know what he asked me to do?" she confessed to Peggy in their nightly phone conversation.

"Trixie, I've told you to be careful out there. You just never know who a person really is," cautioned Peggy.

"I know, honey, but I get so lonely when E.R. is out on his paramedic duties. And if he isn't responding to some emergency, then he's at church or reading that Bible of his. Now, I think everybody ought to go to church on Sunday—after all, why would we all need to get new Easter clothes and such if we didn't go to church? But that man is just obsessed with the Bible. I mean, it is downright obscene how he quotes every little thing and tries to apply it all to me. If you ask me, I think he is just spiritually obese. He calls it Old Testament thinking. I just think it is way too old-fashioned for me. I'm going to stick with just reading the red print in my Bible. You know, those are the true words of Jesus in red, and Jesus don't speak no bullshit, if you will pardon my French."

Peggy had to agree with her cousin to some degree, because there was hardly anything that could get to Peggy faster than someone trying to push their form of religion on her.

There had been a time when Peggy and Troy and their children were regular attendees at church and Sunday school, and Troy had even been a deacon at one time. Peggy couldn't remember exactly when they all began to drift from the Mt. Pisgah Church of Christ, but with Lisa Marie married and Troy Jr. now out of high school and attending vocational school, and Troy, in his words, "getting saved on the golf course" every Sunday, Peggy more often than not avoided suffering through another of Brother Royce's fiery ninety-minute sermons.

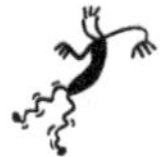

January 28, 2000

-----Original message-------

To: drcarroll@thesexladyonline.com

From: trixielovesvols@yahoo.com

Subject: ONLINE

Dear Dr. Carroll,

Can you believe I am really online? All of us here made it just fine through all that Y2K stuff and I hope you did, too. Oh, honey, this is just so exciting. I am sure you know that our brand-new Tennessee Titans are playing in the Super Bowl. We haven't been this wound up since the Volunteers, bless their hearts, won the national football championship two years ago. Why, honey, every single person in the whole entire state was just going crazy when that happened, so I cannot even imagine what will happen when those Titans bring home the Super Bowl title. I have to go to Kroger's and get some guacamole and chips and some Ro-Tel. It just would not be a real Super Bowl party without Ro-Tel. And do you know what? That Troy is going to fry a turkey in his big old kettle. He's got it all rigged up, and he's even using peanut oil so that turkey won't catch fire while it's frying. I sure hope he knows what he's doing.

Your friend,

Trixie

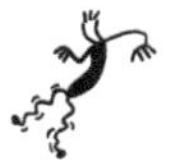

February 5, 2000

To: trixielovesvols@yahoo.com

From: drcarroll@thesexladyonline.com

Subject: Re: ONLINE

Trixie,

I am sorry the Titans lost the Super Bowl. From what I heard, it was a really good game and they were only one yard from the goal line when time ran out. I hope everyone there is not too upset.

I have never heard of a deep-fried turkey. Please let me know how it turned out.

Carroll

Carroll Murphy, PhD, CST, FAAST

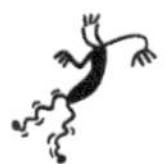

February 8, 2000

To: drcarroll@thesexladyonline.com

From: trixielovesvols@yahoo.com

Subject: Re: Re: ONLINE

Dear Dr. Carroll,

Thank you for writing. My little old heart is almost broke after that ball game, but I just have to pick myself up and keep on going. Rainey—she's my mama, but you probably remember that—anyway, she always tells me you can't see where you're going if you keep looking back behind you, but it sure is hard to keep from wanting them to have just one more play so they could score.

Anyway, thanks for writing me back. I think I will really like having this computer and being online. E.R. claims the Internet is the invention of the devil, but here in Tennessee we all know Al Gore really invented it.

Your friend,

Trixie

P.S. Troy's deep-fried turkey sure was good. And nobody caught on fire!

P.S.S. T. Roy—that's Peggy and Troy's boy—he decided to give himself a highfalutin' name now that he's not a teenager anymore—he says he is going to open himself up a little stand outside those Titan games and deep fry Moon Pies for all the tailgaters. What will they think of next?

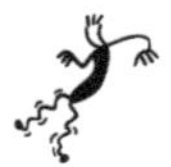

February 21, 2000

Nashville

It was fairly unusual for Trixie and Peggy to have the same day off. The Beautique Salon and Day Spa was open for business Tuesday through Saturday, and the colonoscopy clinic operated Monday through Thursday, but with President's Day being celebrated on the third Monday of February, Peggy also had the day off.

"Let's meet at the Bongo Java coffee shop," Peggy suggested when she phoned her cousin on Sunday night.

"Bongo what, honey? I don't believe I have ever heard of that place."

"It's the one over by Belmont University where they have that Nun Bun. You know, the cinnamon bun that came out looking like Mother Teresa, and then they shellacked it and put it on display. It's made the national news."

Nashville had lots of unusual attractions, from the world-famous Upper Room mural at the United Methodist headquarters to the downtown warehouses that had served as houses of ill repute during the Civil War when Nashville had more prostitutes per capita than any other American city, to the statue of Athena in the Parthenon. But the Nun Bun was a unique treasure.

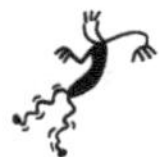

"Lord, honey, it does look like that nun. I can see why she wouldn't have wanted people wearing a T-shirt with a picture of this bun on it. She really needed to get some Botox for those wrinkles."

Trixie looked around the coffee house and wondered about their safety in the midst of the variously garbed students. She was particularly wary of the young man at the next table, whose tattoos and pierced tongue made her squirm.

"Trixie, I don't think that's why she objected. I think she thought it was just not right to associate her image with something like this."

"Whatever," Trixie rolled her eyes and ordered a double latte.

"Well, I declare," she exclaimed, scrunching up her face as she tasted her drink. "Why in the whole wide world would people want to drink something what tastes like this and costs so much, when you can just perk your very own Maxwell House in your own kitchen and then put anything you want in it? But, honey, some people have more money than they have sense and it wouldn't surprise me one little bit to hear they're putting these coffee places on every corner of every city in this whole country."

Peggy nodded. It had been less than three months since Starbucks had opened its first Nashville franchise.

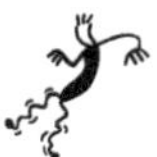

April 13, 2001

-----Original message-------

To: drcarroll@thesexladyonline.com

From: trixielovesvols@yahoo.com

Subject: Trollops

Dear Dr. Carroll:

Thank you so much for asking how the Trollops are coming along. You just won't believe what a good time we are having in our club meetings. And I am learning so much. Why, honey, last night we met at LaDonna's house and Lord, wouldn't you just know she and Crystal had decided they would just surprise us all and put on one of those Passion Parties. Well, honey, I never in this whole wide world ever knew there was such a variety of sex toys out there. It was just like being at a Tupperware party. Well, I didn't buy anything to take home, since I knew it wouldn't do any good in my bedroom, if you get my drift, but some of those girlfriends left there with their arms just full.

But anyway, honey, here's what I really wanted to tell you. Do you remember how I told you on the airplane about Peggy and me starting an Oprah Book Club back here right about the same time as we started our Trollops Sorority? Now, as you know, Peggy and me were going to keep things under our hat about the Trollops and all because we didn't want just every Tom, Dick, and Harry—or I guess in this case it would be every Jane, Beth, and Mary (Ha, ha)—to catch wind of us. You know, honey, there are some people in our neck of the woods, bless their hearts, who just might not understand what we are about, and they might get their noses all out of joint and cause a big old fuss if they thought we were trying to say we thought it was a good thing for some girls to get pregnant before they're married. I mean, we're not trying to promote loose behavior or anything, but we—I mean Peggy and Joan—well Joan's still in Michigan but we tell her every single thing what happens—and Rainey and the others and me, well, honey, we just thought we could have some fun, being that we were a sisterhood and all. Now, I told Rainey about the Trollops right soon after we got home from Virginia because, well, she just sniffs everything out anyway and, honey, do you know what she said? She just up and told me she guessed she could qualify as a charter member herself, thank you very much, so then she started coming to some of our Trollops meetings, and she even invited her best friend, Ella, and before long, well we had about as many senior citizens as we had us middle-aged ladies. To tell you the truth, Dr. Carroll, you could have knocked me over with a feather when Rainey told me about being a charter member, 'cause since I am her one and only child, that makes me a almost illegitimate baby. But then, I guess that's why she got so upset about me having Calvin so prematurely back then.

Well, things were going about as good as anybody could expect. I mean, having two meetings a month to go to and all—one being the Trollops sorority and the other being the Music City A-list Book Club—kept us pretty busy, but as far as I could tell, everybody was just having so much fun it didn't really matter, and Rainey and the senior citizens, well they didn't go to the A-list meetings. They said they were done with reading anything except Danielle Steele books, and we don't ever have those books for the book club. Whatever. Anyway, lo and behold, one time about a year ago, why just out of the blue at the A-list meeting, I blurted out about going to the Trollops meeting the week before and what fun we'd had, and some of those A-list girls, well, they wanted to know what I was talking about, and before you know it, I had spilled the beans. And Dr. Carroll, can you believe it? Right then and there we had five more new members sign up for the Trollops! And then, after a few more months, the rest of the A-list girls, well, they wanted to be Trollops, too, and we said "sure" because, after all, we're easy, and then pretty soon we had just merged the whole shebang. When I told Joan about all of this, she said we should just call ourselves the Music City Trollops A-list Book Club, so that's what we did. So there you have it. Nowadays there are about twenty of us in the sorority, and sometimes we discuss books and sometimes we just have fun, but it doesn't matter one bit to me.

Your friend,

Trixie

P.S. I still tell E.R. I am just going to my book club meeting, and he says I sure have taken an intellectual turn in my old age.

P.S.S. And do you know what else? There is another chapter of the Trollops what has formed right here in Music City and they call themselves the Bawdy Broads because they are the Beta chapter, whatever that means.

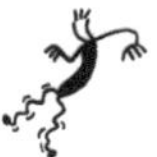

Carroll could visualize the latest headline in the *Enquirer*: TROLLOPS SORORITY MORPHS INTO BOOK CLUB! *I wonder what E.R. would say if he read that.*

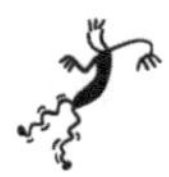

May 7, 2001

Southern California

"So they still have you hooked, huh, Carroll?" Dr. Sutton inquired as he and Carroll sat in his office, discussing her latest research efforts on behalf of the Tennessee Trollops.

"Oh, Dr. S. Please don't say it that way. I know you think it's my counter-transference issues, but I honestly think I may be the only source they have for good information."

"Really? From what you have said, Peggy—the nurse—is getting her master's degree, so don't you think she is capable of figuring some things out for them without your help, Carroll?"

"Yes, I agree, but Trixie doesn't want to bother Peggy with this, since she is finishing work on her thesis and working full-time too."

"Oh." He drew a long breath on the empty pipe, and his eyes twinkled above his half-rims. "So, it's perfectly okay to bother Dr. Carroll, since she doesn't have anything else to tend to, is that right?"

"I guess there is some truth to that. But here—let me read you what Trixie wrote this week." Carroll opened her briefcase and pulled out Trixie's latest e-mail.

"Honey, you won't believe this, but Frank says he thinks he got AIDS from hookers what work the truck stops across the country. He absolutely swears he has never done the deed with a man or that he has used I.V. drugs, and I believe him. There's not much about him I do believe, but he was as much against gays as E.R. is—though for different reasons—and he always said his best friend, Jack Daniel, was the only thing he needed to put in his body to get a high, so I think on this subject he is telling the truth."

"So what did you do then, Carroll?"

"I searched the National Library of Medicine Web site, then I answered her. Here, read this." Carroll handed Dr. Sutton a copy of her e-mail response.

"Trixie, I think you are correct. Frank perfectly fits the profile of a trucker who has unprotected sex with a number of women, and we know right now in this country there is an epidemic among this group of people. I am so sorry you and your family are having to go through this situation."

"Well, I will say one thing, Carroll. You are getting so you can write your friends a paragraph and not a textbook. Good job."

Carroll smiled. For once, he hadn't probed her motives.

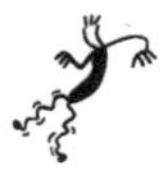

September 16, 2001

--------Original message------

To: drcarroll@thesexladyonline.com

From: trixielovesvols@yahoo.com

Subject: 9/11

Dear Dr. Carroll:

We are just so upset here I don't hardly know what to do. Who would have thought those nasty Arab boys would get in those big old airplanes and run them smack dab into those buildings? I just cannot believe that thousands of little children are waking up every morning now without their daddies or their mamas because of this. Oh, Dr. Carroll, I got me one of those red, white, and blue ribbon pins and then Rainey had to have one, too, and now she has mounted a United States flag on her walker, and Floyd has gotten her a *United We Stand* bumper sticker for her basket, and she says she is going to go protest at the Al Menah Shrine Temple right in downtown Nashville. Now Calvin told me they are not really Arabs down there, even if they do wear those funny hats and such, so I told her she'd better just stay put right at home. For somebody what's almost eighty years old, she sure can keep up with things. I hope you are not being run completely ragged with people calling you or coming into your office with all this mess.

Your friend,

Trixie

P.S. E.R. has been at work for five whole days. They put all emergency personnel on 24/7 alert, and I haven't seen hide nor hair of him since 9/11. He's bound to be plumb wore out when he finally gets relief.

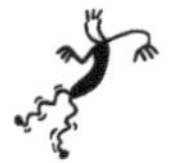

September 17, 2001

Southern California

Carroll was surprised to find the freeways relatively uncrowded as she made her way to Dr. Sutton's office. *Guess some folks are still staying home. Cocooning, they're calling it.*

"Hi Carroll. I'm glad you got here today. I got your message about being stranded in Chicago."

Carroll accepted his requisite cup of tea and walked to the outside deck at his office, which overlooked the Pacific. The crashing of the waves and barking of the seals had always been soothing for Carroll, but today she felt no comfort.

"I'm a mess, Dr. S. I haven't slept more than an hour or two since all this happened. First of all, everybody back here was falling apart, and I must have run up hundreds of dollars in phone bills just trying to handle all their crises from afar. Then the show asked me to do several tapings, since they couldn't get any of the regularly scheduled guests to Chicago without planes flying. But the worst part is the nightmares have come back worse than ever. I'm just worn out."

She leaned forward, letting her head drop between her legs, and her hair flew in all directions across her knees. Sitting back up, she gathered the errant curls into a hank and twisted it, securing it with a chopstick, which she produced from her purse.

Catching Dr. Sutton's questioning eye, she said, "I know I look awful, but I just don't care at the moment."

"Carroll, I think you'd better tell me more about the nightmares."

She sighed and drew in another breath, then slowly began to speak.

"Well, as usual, I was Shirley Temple, dancing and smiling and waving to a crowd, when someone suddenly snatched me up and carried me up above the clouds. Dr. S., I know these dreams are dissociative episodes. I think it must have to do with going to see *Heidi* when I was about seven years old. I remember when Heidi's aunt came and took her away from her grandfather, I cried and cried."

"Yes, that makes sense, and of course you and half the world have been triggered by what happened last week, but I think it must be something more than the movie that set you up for these nightmares, for you still to be having such a reaction today—more than forty-five years after you saw it. It makes me think something else must have happened involving dancing and loss. What comes to mind when I say this to you?"

Dr. Sutton's kind eyes and white beard could have been scripted right out of *Heidi*, and Carroll always was surprised she let herself open up a little more to him than she did to anyone else.

"Well, I was at my dance recital when my father died, but I think I'm over it now," Carroll volunteered without emotion.

"We'd better talk about it, Carroll," Dr. Sutton said.

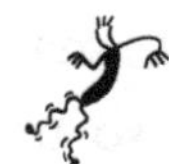

1952

Art Murphy loved his daughter with a fierceness that sometimes frightened his wife. Watching her husband patiently teaching little Carroll to ride her bicycle or to roller skate, while he balanced his athletic body on his one good leg, Frances would glimpse traces of the little boy she had never known. After they married, Art rarely spoke of his childhood, and when he did, his eyes clouded and got a faraway look that was impossible for Frances to fathom. As a nurse, she had seen the same look in the eyes of numerous soldiers who never spoke of the wartime horrors they had witnessed. In fact, the only way she could really know when Art got stuck in his never-ending loop of terror was when she would hear him cry out in his sleep and then bolt upright in their bed. He would slip out from the covers, grab his crutches, and thump barefoot across the room to his chest-of-drawers in the corner, where his ever-ready unfiltered Camels would offer the temporary solace he needed to get through the night.

Carroll would often awaken, too, hearing her dad's shuffle as he moved across the bare wood floor. Somehow it was reassuring to smell the tobacco, as its fragrance made its way to her nose. She would lie in the adjoining room under the chenille bedspread in her high twin bed and pick at the thread balls that ran in neat rows from one end to the other of the cover. By the time she was six years old, the spread had been turned upside down and back and swapped with the one on the other bed, as her mother tried to even out the damage, but Carroll always managed to find another row of little cotton balls to worry off.

The dresser top of their mahogany bedroom suite was scarred by cigarette burns in so many places Frances could no longer conceal them with doilies and ashtrays. Even though Art was barely thirty years old, his fingers had grown yellow from their daily contact with the nicotine, and he had begun to cough with almost any exercise. Always fit, he now had difficulty crossing a room, and more often than not, he could not finish coaching his high school football team's games without having to sit.

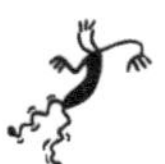

At not quite eighteen, Art joined almost all of his teenaged peers and enlisted in the Army the day after Pearl Harbor. He was sent to the European front, and two and a half years later he was in a Higgins boat in the third wave of the Normandy invasion, coming ashore at Omaha Beach. Nothing could have prepared him for the gruesome scene he encountered that early June afternoon.

Up to that point in his life, Art associated beaches with summer jobs and fun places near his home on the Jersey Shore, where he started out as an umbrella boy and progressed to dressing room attendant and finally to life guard. He anticipated graduating from high school in June of 1942, and had planned to go on to Warfield University, which had tentatively offered him a football scholarship. Most of the people in his high school did not understand why he wanted to go to such a college. His ball-playing buddies from high school were going on to schools like Delaware or Penn State or some other northeastern university, but to Art the opportunity to play ball in the Southeastern Conference seemed like a dream come true.

As Art made his way across the hundreds of bodies of his brethren that June afternoon and ascended the bluff where so many had already fallen under the assault of the German guns, he stopped and vomited one more time. He had not eaten since early morning, when the soldiers were fed full breakfasts of eggs and sausages, but he and his comrades had been nauseated by the choppy waters of the English Channel, turning the floors of the cramped invasion boats into virtual seas of putrid slime. There was nothing left in his body to retch out, but the nausea had not stopped, and he heaved bile into the upturned helmet of a dead lieutenant.

Art's unit was almost completely wiped out during the assault on the beach, but he managed to join up with the tattered remnants of other units which eventually became part of the larger, regrouped force that battled across France on their way to liberate Paris. Before his group reached Paris, Art stepped on a land mine and his left leg was blown off just below the knee. A buddy knotted his bandana around the ravaged stump, slowing the blood loss to a trickle. Art lost consciousness and awakened much later in an American army hospital in England, with the face of an angel looking down at him. Her name was Frances.

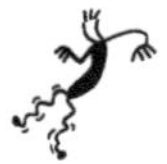

Art's recovery was slow and tedious, and it was more than a year before he and Frances saw one another again. In December of 1945, with the war over and Frances back in the States working in the emergency department at Cook County Hospital in Chicago, Art traveled to the Windy City for a reunion with the nurse whose angelic eyes had met his in those bleak days after his injury. Art's tanned and muscular body was still apparent in his knit shirt and khaki trousers with the left lower pants leg carefully tucked up. Even using crutches, his athleticism impressed Frances. By the end of their first real date, both of them knew they would marry and they did so one month later in a small service in the hospital chapel, attended only by Frances's sister and Art's bunkmate from the Army hospital.

The amputation ended Art's future as a football player in the Southeastern Conference, but it did not stop him from his dream of a college education. Like thousands of other recently discharged servicemen, he found the means to get his education through the GI Bill. He and Frances stayed in Chicago, where her nursing career flourished, and he completed his degree in history at the University of Chicago. A natural-born coach, he volunteered to coach high school football in their neighborhood while he was still in college. The players at first were skeptical they could learn anything from a one-legged man on crutches, but it took only a few practices for Art's love of the game and his talent with his throwing arm to win them over.

He was recruited by several high schools in the area as a history teacher and coach, and at the age of twenty-eight, Art

Murphy was a local legend for his ability to turn relatively untalented teens into winning teams. He and Frances bought the house of their dreams in Evanston and settled down with their only child. One crisp afternoon in the fall of 1952, Art bumped through the back door, using his crutches to alternately push and pull a huge box containing a first-edition black Weber kettle grill, which he promptly assembled. He fired up the charcoal to grill a steak and smiled with great satisfaction. He always liked being the first in the neighborhood to have a new gadget.

"I'm really home," he declared. Frances hugged their little daughter and squeezed his hand as a tear slid down her cheek. At that moment life seemed really good after the hell they had been through.

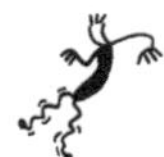

Carroll didn't know where Korea was or what a hydrogen bomb was, but she could tell that the grownups whose conversation she monitored on Saturday night as they played bridge on the kitchen table of her parents' tidy Evanston home, were concerned about both. She noticed the men at the bridge table almost always paused in their trumping or bidding to light another cigarette when certain topics came up. In her six-year-old mind, words like *Japs* and *vaporization* seemed to be written in the smoke above their heads, like she'd seen a few months earlier from the skywriting airplane her dad had taken her to see on her birthday. Art said cheese and snapped her picture with his new Brownie camera in front of one of the planes. She helped her mother put the ruffle-edged photo in her scrapbook, carefully tucking the corners under black edge frames, which she licked and stuck to the paper.

Carroll was not naturally athletic like her father. Art balanced her on the seat of her new bike and started her down the sidewalk with the reminder to "keep pedaling and don't look back." Her face became very serious, her brow furrowing and her tongue lapping the edge of her upper lip, until it found its niche just to the right of center, where it stayed firmly put throughout her endeavor. More often than not, Carroll's intense concentration was broken by a wobble, then a crash, as the bike ran off the sidewalk into a light pole or a neighbor's garbage can. Frances would look out from the front porch to see her husband leaning his crutches up against the offending bike, while he comforted his precious redheaded daughter. He never criticized or gave up on her, as so many of his contemporaries might have done. In Art's mind, Carroll could do anything she put her mind to.

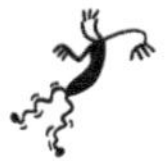

January 14, 1953

"We have to get going," Frances urged, but Art was determined to have a photo to commemorate his daughter's first dance recital. It took him only a few minutes to thread the new roll of film in the Brownie, which he then handed to Frances. He took Carroll's hand in his and balanced on his one good leg in front of the brick fireplace in their tidy home. Remembering his fierce pride, Frances moved his crutches out of range of the camera's viewfinder. Carroll was wearing her black patent tap shoes and the green velvet shorts and pink satin top that Frances had carefully sewn. She kept trying to rein in her tongue, which wanted to taste the lipstick her mother had just dabbed on. Frances was a little unsure of herself operating Art's newest gadget, but he assured her that anyone could be an amateur photographer with this new camera. Before the shutter clicked, Carroll heard both of her parents say "Cheese."

As the children were preparing to march in line onto the stage, their dance teacher reminded them to "S-M-I-L-E, smile, no matter what happens." Carroll was smiling so hard her jaw ached. The troupe was nearing the end of their first segment when she noticed a commotion in the audience. The dancers continued their routine through the shuffle-step-back step-rock-step-point-step, even when the music on the amplified phonograph stopped playing. The heavy velvet curtain quickly closed around some of their small bodies before they saw it coming, and a few of them began to whimper and cry. Carroll kept dancing and smiling even as she was being enveloped. Several parent helpers herded the little dancers offstage to the dressing room, where most of the parents quickly bundled their children out the door, shushing their questions as they glanced back at Carroll.

Midge Rubens, her best friend's mother, found Carroll standing alone in the hallway. "I'm sorry, honey. I have to drive you home. Your mother's gone to the hospital where they took your daddy. Janie's daddy drove her there in your daddy's car. You get in the back seat of our car, and Janie can sit in the front seat with me."

Midge handed Carroll her coat to put on over her dance costume. Carroll could hear the tap-tap-tap of her shiny black patent shoes as they brushed the sidewalk with each step on that unseasonably warm Chicago night. As she sat in the back seat of the Buick sedan, she fingered the seam in the fake leather seat cover and wondered if she might be able to hear the air flow from Janie's mother's Dynaflow, which was all the rage among car buyers that year. Her dad often told her a Buick would be their next car, "just as soon as I buy your mother a fox throw for her shoulders," he said. Somehow, as her ears strained to hear the flow of air, she knew neither of these things would ever happen now.

The house was dark when they got there, but Carroll knew where they kept the secret key in the backyard. She easily opened the back door into the kitchen and flipped on the kitchen light. Midge and Janie followed her in, and the girls sat down at the table. Midge reached into the refrigerator for a glass of milk for each of them. Janie downed hers in one gulp, but Carroll just slowly turned her glass in a circle, feeling the cold, wet condensation rubbing onto her fingers.

Frances came in looking red-eyed and frazzled shortly afterwards, followed by Janie's dad, Howard. As soon as she saw her dad, Janie jumped up and hugged him, holding on tightly while Howard encircled her bony shoulders with his strong left arm. Howard shook his head to answer Midge's questioning eyes, and Frances sat down with Carroll at the red-topped kitchen table with its shiny chrome legs. Carroll had loved rubbing her hands up and down the cool chrome when she was younger, listening to the after-dinner conversation between her parents.

She had never before seen her mother with such a vacant look in her eyes.

With the straightforward, piercing gaze that had characterized her since she was a toddler, Carroll demanded of her mother, "Where's Daddy?"

"Your daddy's gone, honey," Frances answered.

"Gone? Where?" she asked. "Has he gone to Korea? Has he been vaporized? Why won't you tell me where my daddy is?"

Frances Murphy stood and opened the high cabinet above the refrigerator and lifted out a long-necked bottle with a black label on it. She poured the liquid into a double old-fashioned glass that she removed from the cabinet next to the sink, and as she raised the glass to her lips she looked around their warm kitchen. Carroll did not realize it at the time, but she had just witnessed the beginning of her mother's lifelong affair with Jack Daniel.

"He's gone to heaven, honey," her mother gently told her. Carroll didn't believe her. Her daddy had never in her entire life gone off without kissing her and asking, "How's my pal?"

Carroll glared at her mother, who didn't seem to notice, then she bent down and untied the grosgrain ribbons of her tap shoes and threw the shoes in the trash barrel outside the back door, slamming the door loudly behind her. Looking out into the spacious backyard where her swing set sat empty, she spotted the Weber grill, covered with melting snow. She walked over barefoot and kicked it. A cascade of water rushed off into the yard. Her big toe ached, but she ignored it. After all, her mother had always told her to hold her feelings inside because they had to be strong for her dad. He didn't like to see his girls cry. Carroll bit her lip as hard as she could and the tears stayed put.

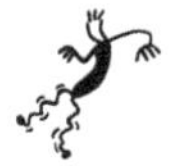

"Maybe there's something there you need to explore further, Carroll," Dr. Sutton said.

"I don't think so. What's over is over. There's nothing to be gained by looking back." Carroll blotted her lower lip, where the tooth mark was oozing slightly, and folded away her pad of note paper. She put her glasses and pen in her briefcase and shook her hair, re-clipping a loose strand behind her left ear.

"See you next week, Dr. S.," she said as she hurried out the door

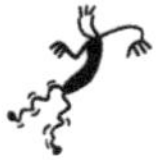

January 25, 2002

——Original message——

To: drcarroll@thesexladyonline.com

From: trixielovesvols@yahoo.com

Subject: Peggy's online

Dear Dr. Carroll:

Oh, you just won't believe this, but Peggy has got herself online. After all this time, when she just pooh-poohed the rest of us who were there in outerspace just having the time of our life, then she went and got herself enrolled in graduate school, and wouldn't you just know, they said they expected all their students to get themselves up to speed on the Internet because that was going to be the future of medicine, and besides all the students would be doing their research on the Web. Now, if that don't beat all.

Well, anyway, honey, I just wanted to let you know one of these days you will probably have two of us Trollops writing you in L.A, and by that I don't mean Lower Alabama. Ha-ha. (L.A.is what my girlfriends have started calling it when they go on their vacations to Gulf Shores, where I have never been and probably will never go.)

Your friend,

Trixie

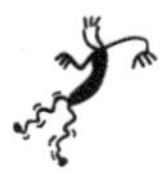

March 2002

Park City, Utah

Mitch Morrissey almost never was sick, but if he did get a cold, especially a nasty one with coughing and sneezing, he had no choice but to temporarily suspend seeing patients in his office. "After all," he would say, "would you want your dentist working in your mouth when he is sneezing all over the place?"

Usually, he could stay in the office and do paperwork when he was sick, and there was enough of that to keep him perpetually office-bound. When he awoke today, however, and there was ten inches of new snow on top of the ice sheet left from the freak early spring thaw and refreeze, he decided to chuck the office routine.

"It's not going anywhere anyway," he always said about the mounds of papers to be pushed or signed as he and all his colleagues coped with the ever increasing regulatory demands on the practice of modern dentistry.

"Isn't it ironic," he would say to his pilot friends with whom he played poker regularly, "the more unregulated the airline industry becomes, the more regulated health care becomes?"

He was mindlessly surfing the channels on his television, when he happened to glimpse Carroll. Her confidence and professionalism caught his attention first, followed shortly by the curves of her cashmere sweater and her flat belly, which he noticed as she sat on Oprah's couch.

Hmmm. Either this is a woman who has never had a baby or she has been in the gym every day of her life toning those abs.

As the camera zoomed in on Carroll, her glowing skin and shining eyes, framed by her cap of auburn tresses, almost took away what little breath Mitch had left in his lungs after being up all night coughing.

"She's the dame that blew me off at Deer Valley!" Mitch nearly shouted at the television. If he hadn't felt so bad, he might have reached out and shaken the screen.

"So, this new study from the University of Chicago says forty-three percent of women are sexually unhappy in their relationships. Why do you think this is so, Dr. Carroll?" asked Oprah.

Mitch sat straight up. He had heard a few of the women who worked in his office mention a sex therapist whom they watched on the Oprah show, but he had never paid much attention to what they were saying.

"Well, if you'll pardon my borrowing a line from one of your late-night colleagues, I think I can illustrate the problems with my *Top Ten Reasons* list," answered Dr. Carroll.

The cameras panned the studio audience, where almost every woman was elbowing her seatmate and nodding enthusiastically.

"Top Ten? Really. How many are on the full list, Dr. Carroll?" and the television hostess turned to stare at the seated guests and the camera. The audience hooted and shouts of "twenty," "fifty," "hundreds," wafted through the studio.

"Let's look at the monitor. I call these my *T's*, since they all start with that letter. Number ten, television. Number nine, trauma. Number eight, testosterone. Number seven, temperament. Number six, tender. Number five, techniques. Number four, tension. Number three, timing. Number two, ticked off. And the top reason I find why most women are not interested in sex is number one, tired."

"Wow! Is that right, ladies? Is this list true for you?" Oprah turned to the mostly female studio audience, where almost all the women were conversing with their companions. The few men in the seats seemed to be trying to find ways to escape their confined spaces, but some looked genuinely puzzled by the list.

"Say more about this, Dr. Carroll."

"Okay—number ten, television. While most guys are surfing the tube, most women are trying to relate to their guy by finding a show in common. More times than not, the closest they will come to a joint program will be a few minutes of an old Western movie or a rerun of *Friends*, and then the guy is off searching again.

"True, ladies?"

"Yes," shouted the audience in unison.

"Number nine, trauma. By the time most women have reached their twenties, they have experienced some form of sexual oppression, like sexual harassment. And this is on top of the estimated one in four women who have been victims of sexual crimes. Feeling like a victim is not conducive to positive sexual expression for most women."

"True again?"

"Yes!"

"The next one should be interesting. We are all hearing a lot about finding a magic pill to boost a woman's sexual appetite," said Oprah.

"Number eight, testosterone. I'm glad you brought that up, Oprah, because more often than not, it's not that the woman has too little testosterone, but that the man's is normally about two hundred times more than a woman's. Neither one is right or wrong. It's just the way nature created us, and except in rare medical conditions, or for some women after menopause, there's nothing that needs to be done to change a woman's hormone level. This is why I personally think there'll never be a magic pill for women like Viagra® is for men."

Mitch was sitting upright now, shouting at the screen.

"Way to go, ladies! Blame it all on the men, as usual. First, we are all just slobs who sit around on our duffs surfing channels, then we oppress and victimize you, now it is our hormones that are out of order and, poor little things, it couldn't possibly have anything to do with you. What a load of bullshit!"

He hit the jump button on the remote. As Clint Eastwood rode across the screen in *Pale Rider*, Mitch again wondered aloud what could have possessed his all-time favorite movie actor to make that so-called relationship film—*Bridges of Madison County*—a few years back.

"That dude should stick with what he does best—true westerns," Mitch pronounced.

Feeling a double sneeze building, Mitch grabbed a handful of tissues from the box next to the couch and hunkered down for another onslaught.

When he and Linda were still married, she might have stayed home from work to tend to him if he were sick during the first few years, but later, as the distance between them grew, there was less and less mothering from her. Even though he occasionally pondered whether their marriage would survive to the twenty-five-year mark, still he was flabbergasted to find her letter sitting on the breakfast table when he returned from his annual goose-hunting trip to Canada in the fall of 1998.

Dear Mitch:

I know you are not expecting to receive this, but I think you will understand where it is coming from. Over the years,

I have hoped we would become closer to one another, but in fact, just the opposite has happened. I don't really think there is any blame on either of our parts, but I have reached the point where I am about to turn fifty, and I have never felt lonelier in my life than I do when I am with you.

As you know, I have always had a circle of girlfriends who have served as my escape and distraction. We have jokingly referred to ourselves as the Ya-Ya Sisterhood and we have been there for each other through thick and thin.

Over the past few years, I have become increasingly closer to Sylvia, and about six months ago we went away together and became lovers. Neither of us had ever anticipated such a thing would happen to us. I for sure had never been attracted to another woman, so I am not sure I am really a lesbian, but I do find in Sylvia's arms a part of me I had never known to exist. I realize you can probably never understand this, and you may be repulsed by the idea of your wife being with a woman, but this is what I want for myself at this stage of my life.

It has not been easy for me to reach this conclusion, and I have shed many a tear about it. I doubt you have any idea how many times I've gotten out of bed after you've started snoring, and I've journalled the night away trying to understand this for myself. But the only understanding I can make of it is that I need to be honest with myself and with you and to give both of us the opportunity to live the second half of our lives in the pursuit of happiness.

So, I'm filing for divorce. I don't want or need anything in the way of a settlement from you. When the house sells, we can split the proceeds. I wish only good things for you in the future.

Lovingly,

Linda

Mitch's fury at Linda was already carefully wrapped up like a cocoon by the time they actually faced each other to discuss the divorce, so she saw only the vaguest hint of his irritation. Over the years, she had learned to read the tiny quivers that would involuntarily kidnap his left eye as the outward sign of his inner pain. For a while he accompanied her to therapy to try work on their struggling marriage, but he huffed out one day, saying the female therapist had formed an alliance with Linda, and he felt ganged up on by the two of them.

Despite Linda's insistence that this so-called alliance had not actually happened and her pleas for him to return to the therapist's office, if for no other reason than to confront the therapist about his suspicion, he refused to darken the doors of a therapist again.

"It's all psychobabble!" he declared before turning on the television and zoning out.

After their divorce—which was really just a formality since he didn't contest it—Mitch decided to reinvent himself by fulfilling his dream of living in the West. He settled in Park City, Utah, which he had visited many times since the early eighties for winter skiing. He found there was an enormous influx of people moving to this picturesque village in the Wasatch Mountains above Salt Lake City. And wherever people lived, there would always be a need for good dentistry.

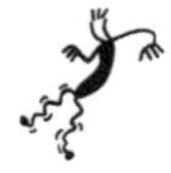

May 19, 2002

Diary entry

Dearest Carroll,

Another Mother's Day has passed. It's the worst day of the year for me in lots of ways. I wish I knew what had come between us that last time you were here, honey. I know you missed your daddy something awful growing up, but I don't think that is why you turned your back on me.

You were always so energetic and so fiercely private that it was almost impossible for me to know what was going on inside you. You seemed to love being on stage—I remember when you played the role of Liesl it was like you actually became her. Everyone who saw you was astonished, and they all expected you to have a movie contract in your future, but you said it was just a phase. I was so surprised when you chose to go to Warfield. You had so many other options, but you said you wanted to complete what your dad had not been able to do.

Do you remember the graduation trip you took to D.C. with Aunt Ann just before college started that fall? You even got to hear Dr. King give his famous speech while you were there. Ann was always such a favorite of yours, and I know you felt like you still had some connection with your dad by being with his sister. I don't know if you kept in touch with her, but, of course, we were devastated when she died of breast cancer a few years later.

I remember driving you down to Warfield. There were not any interstate highways to speak of back then, so it was a tedious ride. The farther south we went, the more quiet you became. I don't think you expected it to be so different from what you had experienced growing up in Evanston, but you never let on if it bothered you. You just stuck out your jaw and moved into that big dormitory where all the girls lived, and, from your letters home, you seemed to be having the time of your life.

You told me you went through rush just to meet people and then you decided not to pledge a sorority. I could understand, because you never wanted anyone else to tell you what to do, and I imagine it would have been hard for you to stick to all the rules if you had pledged.

From the tone of your letters, you seemed to really love your studies at Warfield, particularly the Western Civ class. I remember your glowing accounts of that Dr. Barkley who sometimes had coffee with you after class. Despite all this, I wasn't really all that surprised when you chose to withdraw at the end of your first semester. I thought at the time that the effect of Kennedy's assassination might take a toll on you, and you were pretty quiet when you came home on the train that Thanksgiving. Then at Christmas that year, you got mad at me, and after you went back to finish the semester, we never spoke again. Your terse letter said you were planning on leaving Warfield to move to Oregon and find yourself, and I should not try to contact you. I decided to give you your space, hoping eventually you would turn back to me, but now it has been thirty-eight years and I'm getting to be an old woman, and I don't have much more hope.

I didn't think my heart could ever be heavier than when your daddy died, but I was wrong. It was broken into a million pieces when you left my life. Sometimes I see you today in your TV appearances, looking so confident and obviously loved by your fans, and I wonder if you ever think of me.

You are my precious beloved child.

Love always,

Mother

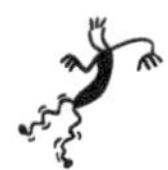

June 4, 2002

Send to: drcarroll@thesexladyonline.com

"Oh, Dr. Carroll, what do you think I should do?" started today's query from Peggy.

Carroll did not hear from Peggy nearly as often as she did from Trixie, and when Peggy did write or do an IM, her queries were almost always to the point, in contrast to Trixie's chatty, rambling e-letters describing some new mess.

There must be something in Nashville's water system that causes all this dysfunction, she thought on more than one occasion.

Once when Carroll remarked about them to Jeanine with whom she shared call, Jeanine described them as the poster children for family messiness. Carroll nodded her agreement.

Thank the Universe I don't have to contend with that kind of family stuff in my own life, Carroll thought. *It's easier being alone.*

Looking back at the scrolling text of the instant message, she read, "Mama is lying up there in that nursing home, thinking she may die before long. God knows, we don't want that to happen, but she says she is bound and determined to die before she turns ninety. She says there is no place in this world for anyone who is over ninety years old. Now I don't know whether that is true or not, but Mama says she can't get buried the way things are."

Carroll looked away from the screen and could imagine what the next sentence would be. Either Mama was not right with God, as was a frequent topic, or else she had gone into another torrent of lambasting Troy for getting Peggy pregnant all those years ago. Mama's short-term memory might not be too good, as Peggy often conveyed, but there was nothing wrong with her long-term memory. And no matter what kind of good works

Troy had accomplished over the years, it could not override in Mama's mind that original sin of his ruining her Peggy.

Glancing back at the screen, Carroll followed along.

"Dr. Carroll, Mama says she is not going to be put in the grave that has been waiting all these years beside our daddy. She says it is not right for a man to be lying there between two wives. No amount of arguing with her will convince her that Daddy didn't have two wives at the same time."

Carroll was a little confused. She had heard part of this story before from Peggy, but it seemed to have had little impact on Peggy's life growing up or as an adult. It was common knowledge that Peggy's father had remarried after a period of widowhood, and there had been no children from the first marriage, and Mama had never voiced any problems with that fact.

Carroll clicked the reply screen. "Are you saying that at almost ninety years old, your mother has suddenly developed an obsession with her deceased husband's also-deceased first wife, who happens to be buried on one side of him?"

"Yes, she is sitting up there in the nursing home telling any and everyone it is just not fitting for a man to lie between two women, and the only way she will go on one side of him when she is buried is if the other woman leaves. And, Dr. Carroll, the other woman has been there for over seventy years, so we can't just go and dig her up and shove her out the door."

As she read this information, Carroll let out a long howl, shouting, "They don't pay me enough to handle these messes."

Grinning, she imagined hearing Dr. Sutton say, *They don't pay you anything for your services*, and she nodded and smiled.

Returning to the screen, Carroll typed, "Peggy, it sounds like your mother is beginning to show signs of aging dementia. This is pretty normal in someone her age, especially if there have been no other signs of true Alzheimer's in her up to now. I think you should ask for the geriatric psychologist in the nursing home to be called to do an evaluation, and see if she might benefit from some treatment."

"Thanks, Dr. Carroll. I'll keep you posted. I hope she doesn't die before we get this worked out."

Peggy

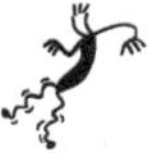

July 3, 2002

--------Original message-------

To: drcarroll@thesexladyonline.com

From: trixielovesvols@yahoo.com

Subject: Elvis

Dear Dr. Carroll:

I hope you won't think we are too weird here in this neck of the woods, but I just don't know where to go to get an answer to this one. Now you know me and E.R. don't exactly see eye to eye about religion. I mean, I think everybody ought to go to church when they can, and Lord knows I have done my share of praying and reading the Good Book over the years, but I just don't cotton to being in church every single little minute that the doors are open. And I'm not sure I would be very good in a missionary position, so to speak, like some of the women from his church, who go out and try to spread the gospel by handing out literature in Walmart and Target. Sometimes I just think a person can get bloated on religion, if you get my drift. Now, not to take anything away from E.R. He's one of the finest men I have ever met and he sure treats me a darn sight better than Frank or Joe ever did, so I am not complaining. But, Dr. Carroll, to tell you the truth, sometimes I think there may be something wrong with him. I mean, I know I am no movie star, but I do think I have held my own pretty well in the age race, but no matter what I do or say or wear or don't wear, that E.R. just does not show any interest in me sexually. I mean, he will give me the tiniest little peck on the cheek, but I practically have to knock him down for that, and he sleeps in a full set of pajamas and just never ever even tries to rub up against me in bed. He claims that since we are not really married—remember I told you we have been living together these past five years, after both of us had had two divorces—well, anyway, he says sex is supposed to be between two married people, and since we are not married, then we should not be having sex. Well, I do think he is right—that is what is supposed to happen, but if a couple chooses not to get married, but they spend all their time together just the two of them, isn't that practically like being married? And what does God think about that? Oh, Dr. Carroll, I know you are not a preacher or anything, but with all those initials after your name, surely you have some ideas about such things. And another thing—Peggy would die if she knew I was telling this to you but, honey, she says Troy has taken to wanting to have Elvis's gospel songs on the CD player when they make love. He calls it the "Church of Elvis Presley," and he gets himself all worked up just hearing that music. 'Course, Peggy has always liked Elvis, too, so she says it doesn't hurt anything either to be imagining Elvis being right there in her bedroom singing those songs.

Now, Dr. Carroll, here's the thing I want to know—do you think I should get a CD of Elvis singing gospel and play it to try to get E.R. warmed up a little?

Your friend,

Trixie

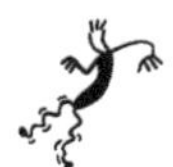

July 5, 2002

To: trixielovesvols@yahoo.com

From: drcarroll@thesexladyonline.com

Subject: Re: Elvis

Trixie—I guess it would not hurt anything to try it. Let me know what happens.

Carroll

Carroll Murphy PhD. CST FAAST

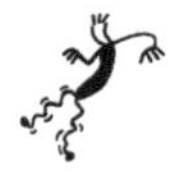

Early October 2002

Southern California

"Dr. S., I won't be able to come for supervision the end of the month. I have to go to Eugene, Oregon to attend a program."

Morris Sutton drew deeply on his empty pipe stem and looked over the rims of his glasses at Carroll.

"Oh, what kind of program takes you into Duck country, Carroll?"

"Well, the U of O Alumni Association has named me as one of the recipients of this year's Distinguished Alumni award and they say I need to be there in person to accept it."

"Sounds like a pretty big deal to me, Carroll. I've never heard you mention much about your time in Eugene, so I find it a little puzzling that you are being honored."

"Well, I did graduate there but like most everything else in my life, once something is over, I put it behind me. I've never been back since 1967, and I almost never read the alumni magazine they send out. But I guess I will go."

"Will you be speaking, Carroll?"

"Yes, I'll give you a copy of my remarks. You always say you don't know very much about me, so this may help you put some pieces together."

"Well, I'll miss seeing you here, Carroll, but I always look forward to learning a little more about you. You are a hard one to fathom."

Dr. Sutton tapped his pipe bowl in the crystal dish on the table next to his chair, and looked across the room at Carroll, who was gathering her things and starting out the door.

"Bye," she said.

"Go Ducks," he responded.

Carroll grinned and closed the door.

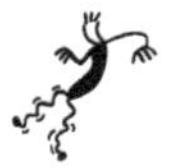

October 14, 2002

--------Original message--------

To: drcarroll@thesexladyonline.com

From: peggybsn@yahoo.com

Subject: Mama's passed

Dear Dr. Carroll,

I don't know whether Trixie has kept you up to speed or not, but I wanted to let you know Mama took a turn for the worst about three weeks ago, and she passed last Friday. We put her in hospice at the end, and she seemed to be real peaceful about it all.

I guess she has stayed put in that grave after all, because when I drove out there today to put fresh flowers on it, it didn't look like anybody had been in a ruckus.

It was hard for all of us to let her go, but she had a good life, and she was ready to go.

By the way, she died one day short of her ninetieth birthday. Isn't that something?

Peggy

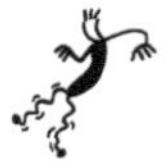

October 20, 2002

To: peggybsn@yahoo.com

From: drcarroll@thesexladyonline.com

Subject: Re: Mama's passed

Dear Peggy,

I am so sorry to hear about the loss of your mother. I know she was really special to all of you, and I'm sorry I didn't get a chance to meet her. Take good care of yourself.

All the best,

Carroll

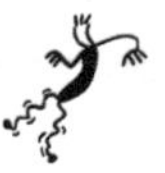

October 25, 2002

Homecoming Weekend

Eugene, Oregon

"Ladies and gentlemen, I am especially pleased to introduce to you the second of this year's recipients of the Distinguished Alumnus Award, Dr. Carroll Murphy. Dr. Murphy is well-known to many of you as America's sex lady from her many appearances on daytime and evening talk-shows where she is often the authority for whatever is the newest sex scandal of some celebrity. She is also a frequent guest on Oprah's show, where millions of women—and quite a few men—enjoy hearing her take on everyday sexual problems.

Listen with me as I read from her citation on this year's award:

'Dr. Murphy is recognized for her outstanding work in the field of human sexuality, where she has pioneered both in her scholarly writings, most recently *The Naked Truth about Lady Godiva*, which was on the best-selling list of the *New York Times* for 58 consecutive weeks, and her media presentations about all areas of human sexual behavior—and misbehavior. At the same time, she has maintained a private practice in sex therapy in Southern California, and she serves as a consultant and instructor to several universities in the area.

Carroll Ann Murphy entered the University of Oregon as a special student in the spring of 1964 and graduated Phi Beta Kappa as one of the Honors College Senior Six top students in 1967. Her interest in human sexuality began during the spring term in 1965 when she was one of 16 students who joined an informal discussion group on their sex problems and their ideas about sex. This lead to an expanded program for the Fall '65 term, aimed at freshmen, with the goal of enlightenment about sex problems and about sexual adventures of college students.'

And, as the saying goes, the rest is history. Please welcome Dr. Carroll Murphy."

As the alumni audience thundered their applause, Carroll reached inside herself and grabbed her actress persona, pasting it over the scared little girl she felt. She stood and received a hug and handshake from the alumni president and acknowledged the other award recipient who shared the stage with them. She placed her prepared remarks on the stand, sipped a drink of water from the glass handed to her, and cleared her throat. Positioning her glasses on her nose, she began to speak.

"Mr. President, alumni, and my fellow recipient, it is indeed an honor to receive this award from my alma mater. This has been my first opportunity to return to Eugene since I left here in the summer of 1967. Yesterday after I arrived, I had a chance to drive around and I'm amazed at the changes that have taken place here. Back then, Eugene was a sleepy little college town. Today it is not quite a bustling metropolis, but I am told that the student population here at the U of O is the largest of any college or university in the state. As I drove through town I was impressed by the numbers of bicyclists in the streets and the ease with which they seem to be able to get around—a far cry from the days when I feared for my life as I dodged pick-up trucks at every intersection while riding my bike from the dorm to my job and back.

"One thing I noticed hasn't changed is Skinner's Butte—it's still smack-dab in the center of town and while lots of trees have matured and you can't see the mansion so well now, the O is still there on the side of the butte—and so is the cross up above it. I grew up in the Midwest and I arrived here on a bus in early 1964 completely unaware of anything about the Pacific Northwest. I spent my first semester in another college and was on the rebound when I landed here. I didn't know what a duck was except for being a waterfowl back then. That was the wettest winter in the history of the Pacific Northwest and with all the rivers and streams flooding, I remember thinking a duck was an appropriate name for a water-logged college to name its mascot. The first time I saw that huge O on the butte, I couldn't imagine what it stood for. Now I know that it's one of hundreds of hillside letters all over western states—though there are none others that represent the Ducks—but I was a letter virgin back then—and I'll always remember my first one."

The audience howled, hearing a typical Sex Lady one-liner.

"On a serious note, I used to look at that cross, lit up by its neon lights, and feel conflicted. I would think, 'why is the city of Eugene displaying a symbol of Christianity in its public park in a time when public entities are supposed to not promote one religion over another.' But I remember somehow also feeling comforted by the cross when I was alone here over Christmas holidays. I must admit, seeing it still there on the butte, I still feel conflicted about its presence.

"When I look back on my U of O experience, I see the time was incredibly pivotal for me both personally and professionally. The three-plus years I spent as a student here were a representative microcosm of changes taking place across America in the mid-1960's. I entered school in the aftermath of Kennedy's assassination, when college students were still pretty apathetic about politics and society in general. By the time I graduated, U of O students—as well as students everywhere—were involved in peace demonstrations; we fasted and demonstrated to protest racial inequalities; we joined faculty in protests against censorship of academic freedom; we were active, aware, sympathetic, and committed. In short we became revolutionaries. And things have never been the same since, thank goodness.

"I changed a great deal myself during those nearly four years. I entered here feeling lost and needing a new start on life. I knew I was bright and I was willing to work hard, but I had no idea what I wanted to do as a career. It was in those informal discussion group meetings about sex on college campuses that I found my passion was working with sexual issues. I loved connecting with incoming freshmen to try to intervene early on in their choices about their sexual behavior, particularly in relation to sex and drinking. Back then hardly anyone would discuss such things in public—although there was no hesitation to discuss them in dorm rooms—and I determined that somehow I would find a way to bring these issues to the forefront and to be a role model for others—both men and women—who struggled to make sense of their sexuality and sexual concerns.

"By the time I graduated, I had become a feminist, although that movement was just beginning to take shape, and I had developed the seeds for my still mostly liberal viewpoints. I could not—cannot—abide people hiding behind stale rhetoric to defend values that were outdated at best, and unhealthy at worst. I enjoyed speaking out for those who had no voice and making uncomfortable those who glorified in their comfort based on separation from their fellow humans. Looking back from this vantage point, I can see all those values of mine started to grow here at the University of Oregon and I am thankful for the experience and the lessons I learned.

"I do have a couple of disappointments about my time here. Since I had no family to support me then, I worked full-time to pay for my expenses while also going to school fulltime. That didn't leave me much time for socializing, but I was able to graduate on schedule (not like some of today's students who are on the extended plan). Looking back, I regret I left behind undeveloped relationships with fellow students. I never had my photo taken for any student publications, and unless a person knew where to look, you would be hard-pressed to find a public record that I was ever here, but I can assure you, I was here. And the University of Oregon receives all the credit for starting me on the road to where I am today."

Carroll took a sip of water and removed her glasses, smiling to her audience as if the TV cameras were rolling.

"I have a confession to make—I'm also a football game virgin—at least a Ducks football virgin. I never went to any games while I was here. I worked in a bar part of my sophomore year—that's back when they didn't check ID's very carefully for drinking ages, especially among servers—and I remember the tears spilled in customers' beers that November night in 1964 when everyone thought the Ducks were headed to the Rose Bowl, and then along came the Beavers. It seemed like the winter floods were starting all over again, I can tell you. Well, I understand the Ducks are doing better these days—won last year's Civil War, I'm told—so I'm looking forward to losing my football virginity later today in front of thousands of folks when the two schools meet again. Go Ducks!

"Many thanks for this award—and thanks for the memories."

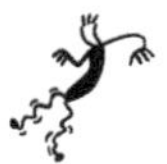

Sunday October 26, 2002

Front page photo, Eugene newspaper, with accompanying headline

"'Sex lady,' Dr. Carroll Ann Murphy, University of Oregon alum class of 1967, one of two honored as Distinguished Alumnus—draws standing ovation for her remarks."

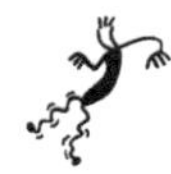

January 13, 2003

Diary entry

Dearest Carroll,

I almost can't believe I am 81 years old. I have been sober for eleven years now, and they have been good years in many ways. You'd be very surprised, I think, to see what I can do on the Internet. Since I never really learned to type, I didn't think I could find my way around online, but I started taking genealogy classes at the Senior Citizens Center, and now I am researching both my family and your dad's. What a miracle the Internet is! I have compiled what I know in a ged.com file, and it's accessible through the Web. Who knows, maybe someday you will look up Art Murphy and find it.

I had both loved and feared Mother Murphy, the name Art used to introduce his mother to me as his new wife when we visited her in New Jersey after our wedding. During our first year of marriage, I never heard Art refer to his mother as anything other than Mother, so I had almost forgotten that his mother was indeed named Carroll, which had been shortened to Carrie when she was a child. I thought the name was lovely, and I especially liked that the spelling reflected the family roots in Scotland, from where Carrie's parents had emigrated in 1900 as newlyweds. So when you were born, you instantly became Carroll. Your dad sometimes shortened it to Carrie but you would insistently correct him—"I do not have a nickname," you would say with your little mouth firmly set and your eyes stern. Calling you Carrie was about the only thing your father could do that you did not adore. And I think he just did it to see you respond.

You so much took after his side of the family—from your hair to your eyes and your Ivory Soap skin, with just a hint of freckles. Everyone on my side was so fair-skinned that any exposure to sunlight would just about ruin us, but somehow your skin just got more beautiful with a tan. Of course, back then we did not know how dangerous the sun could be, so I often wonder if you have ever had any skin cancers. I guess it is the nurse in me to worry about such things.

You are my precious beloved child.

Love always,

Mother

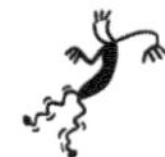

January 24, 2003

Park City, Utah

Mitch had already covered most of the runs at the top of Bald Mountain and was ready for lunch. *I'll be top to bottom in less than two minutes with any luck*, he thought.

He skied off the Homestake Lift and adjusted his boots, grabbed his poles, and dropped down his sunglasses on his nose. Looking up the mountain behind him to make sure the coast was clear, he pushed off past the Solid Muldoon sign to skim the first little hill below him. The morning had been brilliantly clear, with the temperature in the high teens and hardly any wind, but over the last fifteen minutes huge dark clouds had pushed their way along the mountain tops and a fine snow was beginning to fall.

Damn. Getting overcast. Should have brought my goggles.

Cresting the peak, he saw a clot of skiers massed to the left side of the hill, not moving. In front of them were the telltale tracks of a skier in distress—upright crossed poles stuck into the white powder and a loose ski laying uphill from the poles. As he cautiously skied down to the group, he noticed a female figure standing at the edge of the group of onlookers. Down the back of her turquoise ski jacket, a cascade of red hair tumbled over the collar, wet and wild from the shower of snow being deposited on her head.

It's my lucky day! he smirked. *Three long years I've waited to spot that broad again in person. We'll see what she really knows.*

"Dr. Carroll Murphy, I believe," and he bowed to take her gloved hand.

Carroll could have been a frozen ice statue left over from the Winter Carnival a few weeks back. No movement, not even a flinch or a blink. Mitch paused and tried again.

"Hello, remember me? The poor sucker whose pole didn't make it to the top of the lift." Still no answer.

"Anyone home in there?" Mitch questioned, this time waving his hand in front of Carroll's goggled face.

My God, what's the matter with her? She looks like she is in a trance.

He heard the roar of the ski patrol arriving on their snowmobile. Other spectators began to sidestep down the hill, resuming their descent with caution. The lower part of Muldoon was notoriously treacherous, particularly after the sun began to hit it, as it got a little icy when it refroze. Mitch noted that some of the less intrepid skiers were traversing rather than plowing straight down, and for a change he agreed with their method.

Carroll didn't appear to be injured, and one eyewitness confirmed she had been nowhere near the collision. Nevertheless, she seemed to be paralyzed. He had seen this sort of thing happen a few times in his office with patients who got freaked by the sound of a dental drill or the smell of the anesthesia. With them, he had learned, it takes patience—explaining things slowly to get them through their fear.

"Carroll, it's Mitch. Mitch Morrissey. We were on a lift together a couple of years ago. I know who you are from having seen you on TV," Mitch began.

"I'll help you, if you'll let me. You've had a big scare, seeing that woman hit the tree. Carroll, can you hear me? If you can hear, squeeze my hand." He placed his ungloved hand in her gloved one. Feeling a very tentative movement, he asked again.

"I think you squeezed, but I want to be sure. Again, and a little stronger this time, if you can.

"Good, thanks. Now I want to say a couple of things to you. Okay? You can squeeze for yes. If you don't squeeze I'll take it as no."

The squeeze was firm and receded slowly.

"First of all, you're all right. I think you're in shock, though, so I need to get you moving. Lift your feet one at a time."

She picked up each foot about three inches off the ground and set it back down. About thirty seconds of this, and she was actually moving her lower body in a slow cadence.

"Well, it's not exactly Sousa, but I'll accept it as a good imitation of a march," laughed Mitch, whistling the first few bars of *El Capitan* for emphasis.

"Now how about those arms? Anything you can get going there, Carroll?" Her arms remained motionless at her sides.

"Nothing? So . . . I'm going to take hold of one hand and arm at a time and move them around. Here we go."

Her arms moved limply with his assistance.

"Now we have to get you down this mountain and into the lodge. Okay? "

Blinking her eyes, Carroll turned her head slightly towards the male voice and Mitch grinned.

"Atta girl! I knew someone was there behind those Smith goggles. Do you think you can ski down, if I stay right behind you and we traverse very slowly?"

Carroll nodded.

"OK, here we go. You lead the way and we'll take as long as you need to get down."

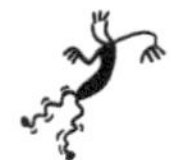

Ten minutes later, they were seated in the lodge at a table by the fire. Carroll's boots were set neatly beside her, and she had her hands wrapped around a mug of coffee.

"Why did you stop to help me, Mitch?" Carroll looked at him solemnly.

"Well, to tell you the truth, my plan was really to hit on you!"

"*Hit* on me?" Carroll blurted, choking on her coffee. Mitch handed her a napkin.

"Thanks." She answered, smiling a little.

The male diners at a nearby table paused in mid-chew. Giving a thumbs-up, one balding guy shouted, "Hey, go for it, buddy!"

Mitch smiled at them and continued. "But it didn't take me long to see you were in no state of mind for that kind of action. And frankly I'm not in to necrophilia, myself."

"Necrophilia?" she sputtered. "Where did you learn that term?"

"Oh, I'm not the only one at this table who took a few psychology classes. Zoophilia, well, that's another story, but definitely no necrophilia."

At the next table, a family with five children looked towards Mitch and Carroll in disgust and rose to begin searching for another place to sit.

Carroll glanced their way and laughed. "Happens all the time when I go to sex therapy conventions. We go out to eat, start talking about cases we've seen, and we can clear a restaurant faster than a tornado siren."

Mitch patted her hand. "It's good to see you laughing. Have dinner with me tonight, will you?"

Carroll hesitated, then nodded. "Okay, but only if we go to Adolph's. I always go there my last night in town, and I've already made a reservation for a table for one. It will be my treat and a way to say thanks to you for your gallantry."

"Agreed." Mitch smiled and shook his head almost imperceptibly, sensing Dr. Carroll was retaking control.

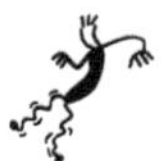

"Carroll, my dear. Lovely to see you again. But who's this handsome young man with you?"

Since the days when his restaurant had been located where the Park City golf pro shop now stands, Adolph had had a special fondness for Carroll. In the new location, the atmosphere and menu remained almost unchanged, full of ski memorabilia and touches of Adolph's home country.

"We have your special table ready, but my dear, we didn't know to expect two for dinner. It will just be a matter of minutes and everything will be set for both of you."

"Thanks, Adolph. This is my friend Mitch. He's a local, but he says this is his first time here."

"Wonderful, wonderful my boy. You are keeping very good company. We love our Dr. Carroll." Adolph's hug for Carroll and handshake for Mitch were lingering and genuine.

Seated in the prime corner booth, Mitch and Carroll watched Adolph return to the kitchen, where he meticulously oversaw every meal that was served.

"When I came here the first time, in about 1983, I was too poor to order anything but dessert. I don't think they had ever had anyone show up requesting a table for dessert only, but the wait staff could not have been nicer to me. I had Bananas Foster and they treated me just like I was paying for the most expensive meal on the menu. I've returned for my last night in town every year since then, and by the 90's I could actually afford the full fare. Now, every time I come in, they automatically prepare Bananas Foster even without my asking. Just wait and see."

Carroll grinned to see their server already preparing the rolling flambé cart for the journey to their table.

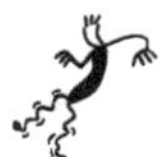

As Carroll and Mitch finished the last bite of their dessert, Adolph rejoined them from the kitchen.

"Ah, it does my heart so much good to see you dining with someone, Carroll. We do love this little lady, Mitch. Take good care of her."

"I will, if she'll let me," laughed Mitch, standing to return Adolph's hug. "I'm learning, though—she's a tough nut to crack."

"Ah, yes, I know what you mean, but those with the hardest shells are always the sweetest ones and worth the patience of getting there."

"As always, Adolph, you know me better than I know myself," Carroll said, standing to hug her Swiss host. The three of them walked together to the front door, and then Mitch and Carroll turned and saluted Adolph as they continued to Mitch's car.

"A finer man I have never known in this town," Carroll said, dabbing at her moistening eyes.

As he pulled his Cherokee out of the parking lot to take Carroll back to her lodging, Mitch asked, "Will you come to my place for an after-dinner drink, Carroll?"

"This is not another come-on—inviting me up to see your Etruscan etchings or something, is it, Mitch?" Carroll asked, grinning.

"Nope, everything's strictly above board, I promise." Mitch winked and patted Carroll's hand.

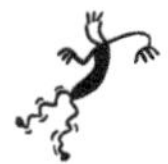

Carroll had expected a drive-in garage followed by an elevator ride, not an outside parking lot filled with snow-covered vehicles and a recently shoveled sidewalk leading to a flight of steps. When Mitch opened the door of his second story apartment for her and flicked on the light, she shivered from the cold she had just left. Mitch's golden retriever, Misty, greeted them at the door, sniffing the new visitor eagerly. Carroll responded civilly but without enthusiasm, and Misty returned to her nap on her pallet near the fireplace.

"Give me a minute and I'll have a roaring fire. I just need to step out on the deck and bring in some firewood," Mitch said.

He was right, and she was feeling much warmer now, sitting on a stool at the raised counter of his kitchen while he pulled out the liqueur glasses. As she looked around, she thought, *For once a guy wasn't exaggerating when he said little cabin.*

She used the tiny powder room adjacent to Mitch's downstairs office, noticing its cleanliness if not exactly its attractiveness. Coming out, she surveyed the rest of the space—a small living room adjoining the kitchen and stairs leading upward. She guessed that was the location of the master bedroom. The apartment was sturdy and functional, but not exactly warm in a decorative sense. *Just like a man. He probably moved in here after his divorce, and once he put everything away, he never gave another thought to accenting it,* Carroll thought.

"How long have you lived here, Mitch?" asked Carroll, watching him carefully pour the bronze liquid.

"Oh, about three years. I didn't really expect to stay put in this apartment when I came to Park City, but it is so inexpensive and convenient that I just never got around to moving anywhere else. I have a cleaning lady who comes in once a week—luckily this was her day—but otherwise I just almost never have anyone here but Misty and me."

Hearing her name, Misty ambled, in hoping for an after dinner treat for herself. She rubbed against Carroll's knees, and Carroll gave her a perfunctory scratch to the top of her head.

"You're not a dog person, are you?" Mitch asked.

"No, I guess not. I don't even have a goldfish!"

"Why not? Don't you like pets?"

"Well, they're okay for other people, but I'm gone a lot, and it doesn't seem fair to leave a pet in an empty condo or in a kennel. Of course, in southern California one can hire a pet nanny to do any and all pet-related chores, but that sort of defeats the purpose, don't you think?

"But do you like pets, Carroll? I mean, sometimes when I come home from work just beat to death with all that I have had to get done there, it's wonderful to have Misty just waiting for me with no grudges from what I did or didn't do yesterday or will do tomorrow. She only lives in this moment, and she thinks I'm the greatest person in the world. That was a new experience for me after my wife left, I can assure you!"

"I don't dislike them, but I don't feel any great attraction for a pet, either. They do seem to comfort many people who have them, and I always recommend them to my clients who have had losses or other disappointments, but I think I'm better off without having a pet."

Carroll accepted the port offered to her in the tiny glass and followed Mitch the few steps into the living room. He offered her a seat in the matching recliner next to his, but she declined, choosing instead to sit on the floor in front of the sofa.

Mitch grinned. *One tough lady*, he thought.

"So you said that your purpose in stopping on Muldoon today was to hit on me. Was that really what you meant to do?"

"My only other purpose was to tell you what a total asshole I thought you were when I saw you on the Oprah show a couple of years ago, telling the world women don't want to have sex anymore because men are such jerks!" Mitch smiled. "Then, when I did see you today, I ended up rescuing you."

"Uh-oh!" Carroll chuckled. "Looks like I stepped on someone's toes."

"No, you didn't step on my toes—and don't start using your psychobabble with me. I'm warning you—I can see through it.

It's just I don't like being blamed for something that is as much a woman's fault as it is a man's, so when you started down your top-ten list, all I could think was 'oh, shit. Another bitch going off on me.'"

Mitch's eyebrow twitched, and he put his finger on it to try to calm the tremulous muscle.

"So why didn't you just call me up or send me an e-mail? Hundreds of others do every day. From the amount of controversy I generate by just talking about what I do for a living, you would think I own the franchise on evil."

Carroll chuckled aloud. It had only been a few months since the current president had been lecturing the world about the Axis of Evil, and she had almost thought he might put her and her profession on his list of threats.

"Because I don't do that sort of thing," Mitch said. "If a person can't face someone directly and tell them what he thinks, I think he is just a coward. So I kept my eyes out for you. You're easy to spot with your red hair, not to mention a body even a blind man could see."

Mitch let out a wolf whistle and Carroll felt her face glowing under the freckles and again she cursed her Scottish heritage.

"So, when you heard me say men could have something to do with women's disinterest, it angered you?"

"Dammit, woman, I told you not to speak psychobabble to me. But, yes, it hurt right smart."

Grinning, Carroll asked, "Did you have a southern mother?"

"What?" Mitch's hands flew up in the surrender position, and his brown eyes stared.

"Well, I don't mean to offend, but that expression—right smart—I believe is one that's often used by people in Appalachia."

"Okay. Yes, my mother did grow up outside of Knoxville, but that has nothing to do with what we're discussing."

Carroll pulled the wool tartan throw she had wrapped around her legs closer, tucking in the end under her Ragg socks. Noticing a little tag on one end of the throw, she turned it up and read, *100% woven in Scotland, Burns Fiber Mill.*

"That's the Grant tartan," Mitch noted. "My grandfather's clan, from the midlands. Do you know anything about your family's background?"

Carroll drew the tartan even closer.

"I don't have any family, Mitch."

"What do you mean you don't have any family? Everybody has a family."

"Well, I don't. At least not any more. I was an only child. My dad died when I was six, and really, my mother died then, too. I was briefly married to Brian. He died when I was in my early twenties. I don't have any children, so I'm completely free to come and go as I please. And that suits me well, thank you very much."

"Did you have a southern mother too?" Mitch asked.

"Why would you ask?" Carroll's startled eyes brimmed with alarm.

"Because the expression—thank you very much—I hear it from the southern women in my practice. There is one thing I have learned about southern women—they learn to speak in code at a young age."

"Well, no, I didn't have a southern mother. But I think my dad's parents grew up in the south. I really don't know much about them. Every now and then when I come here I think about spending a day in the LDS genealogy library researching my ancestors, but then I change my mind and go on and ski. Maybe someday in my old age I'll track them down, but at this point, I really don't care."

The shivers gave way to actual chills. Carroll's trembling caught Misty's notice, and she sidled over from under the table. Her cool, wet nose surprised Carroll.

Misty's uncanny ability to know exactly when to approach and when to stay away from her human charges was the deciding factor in Mitch's bringing her home from the pound with him in the first place, after he and Linda were divorced. More nights than not, Misty slept at the foot of Mitch's bed and was the first to greet him in the morning, her deep brown eyes trained on his.

The fire had died down some, and Mitch reached deep under the embers and stirred with his fireplace poker, then turned to the woodpile and added three more choice logs to the coals. In a minute, they had caught and were adding their warmth to the coolness of the winter night.

He padded to the kitchen to refill his glass, his moccasins flapping against the travertine tiles with each step. "Don't know why they keep putting all this stone and tile in these places, when it doesn't get above freezing nine out of twelve months," he said, turning his head towards the living room.

As he returned, carrying a refill for her, Carroll looked up at him and smiled, then said, "No, thanks. I think I'll stop with one." He set the small glass on the coffee table.

"Okay, maybe I'll drink it for you later on. It's hard to get it back in the bottle."

Carroll grinned, and then fixed her look on the waxing fire.

Minutes passed, and the old-fashioned mantel clock sounded the quarter hour with three chimes. Carroll glanced up at it.

"My grandfather's clock. I inherited it after he passed on. Do you like it?"

"Do I like . . . what?" Carroll asked, looking forlorn. Her rosy face had grown pale, and Mitch feared she might topple into the fireplace.

"Here, why don't you back up and lean into the sofa. Use this pillow."

Carroll gratefully accepted his kindness and again wondered at herself for allowing someone to care for her. She shifted her position and gazed again into the fire.

"On second thought, maybe I'll have that port. I think it might be restorative."

"Sure," Mitch said, smiling, as he handed her the little glass. "So are you going to tell me something about yourself or do I have to get you roaring drunk before you'll open up?"

Carroll whirled around and fixed a furious gaze on Mitch. "Don't ever, ever say such a thing to me again! I mean it. Don't ever threaten me with alcohol."

She sat the tiny glass, still full, back down on the coffee table.

The clocked chimed the hour and Mitch stirred the fire, then sat back down in the recliner and waited for Carroll to go on.

"When I was a little girl growing up, I had to invent lots of ways to make myself seem okay. All of my girlfriends had daddies, except for the one or two whose parents were divorced . . . and at least they got to see their fathers on weekends and holidays. But I felt like something was wrong with me because my father had died." She traced the plaid of the tartan with her index finger, and then absently touched her hair, sweeping an errant curl behind her ear.

"Nobody ever said anything directly to me, but I just felt it—their pity and their judgments. So I invented myself as a super-strong, super-capable person who didn't need anything from anybody. And until today out on the ski slope when you, as you say, rescued me, I have almost never let myself be dependent on anybody."

Mitch listened intently, lifting his port sipper only after Carroll had paused. He drew in the mellow fragrance of the liquid before letting the slightly acid then sweet taste roll over his taste buds and down his throat. With a satisfied *ummm*, he emptied his glass and replaced it with the untouched one of Carroll's.

"Well, that makes sense to me. When I was a boy and my family didn't have some of the things other families had, I just pretended we did have those things, and nobody knew the difference."

"But it was different for me, Mitch. You sometimes didn't have material things growing up. I didn't have parents. Do you know what that's like?"

Mitch shook his head and bent a little closer to Carroll.

"My dad died of a heart attack in front of my eyes while I was dancing in my first recital, and then my mother died slowly over the years as she crawled more and more into her bottle of Jack Daniel's. It was all very respectable, what she did. She was never a public drunk or anything, and the hospital kept promoting her up the ranks, but I was the one who really knew what was going on. It was like I was the mother and she was the acting-out teenager." Carroll paused and dabbed her nose, looking across the table into the fire.

"So, I don't take kindly to the idea of myself being made—what did you call it?—roaring drunk. Believe me, I will do without alcohol before I will ever let myself become intoxicated."

"OK—it was just an expression. But I promise never to say it to you again. Forgiven?"

"Forgiven." She smiled. "Could I have a glass of water, please?"

As Mitch handed her the water, Carroll sighed deeply and continued.

"She would hide her bottles in the clothes hamper. I guess she thought I wouldn't notice them when I was doing the laundry—which I started to do when I was ten years old, because if I hadn't, neither of us would have ever had clean clothes."

The tears fell slowly at first, and then with more rapidity and force.

"I couldn't have any of my girlfriends, and later any boyfriends come over to our house because I never knew what state she would be in. I'm sure they all wondered why I never returned any of their invitations. Some of them probably thought I was stuck up."

She paused and sipped the water.

"All their mothers were amazed at how well my mother managed, but what they didn't know was, for the most part, I did the cleaning and cooking and washing. I spent so much of my childhood parenting my mother that I used to vow never to become a parent myself."

Carroll's shoulders heaved, but when Mitch leaned in to hold her, she shrugged him off, and he pulled back in to the recliner.

"I became an actress in high school, so I could leave my real life beyond the floodlights. I even thought about pursuing a career in the theater, but I knew I needed to do something that would provide more security in the long run. I didn't fool myself or anyone else by thinking I was Oscar material, I can assure you."

She caught his eye, and he smiled.

Odd, the way I'm talking to him like this, she critiqued herself.

"Anyway," she continued, "I had a falling out with my mother when I was home at Christmas of my freshman year, and for me, it was the last straw. At the end of the first semester, I managed to get home to Evanston and pick up my things while she was at work, then I got on a bus to Oregon. I told her never to try to contact me again, and that was the last I saw of her. That was in 1964, so I have been an orphan for almost forty years."

"Forty years is a long time. You seem to have managed quite well, from what I hear of you from the women who work in my office.

"Well, it's all an act, Mitch."

Caught off guard, Mitch drew in a breath and momentarily was speechless.

"An act? What do you mean? You are not the world's greatest sex therapist, the mistress of all media, the queen of the TV talk shows, and a match for even Bill O'Reilly. Yes, I saw you handle him in exactly the same castrating manner that you used on me in our first meeting, but that's okay. I think he needs someone to take him down a notch or two."

Carroll reached for the tissue Mitch had offered. She was glad his favorite brand was the kind infused with lotion.

"If people really knew who I am, they'd see I'm not a very nice, compassionate person. I've created that persona because it sells well and because it's what my clients expect, but it's not who I really am."

"Well, who the hell are you, then?" Mitch asked, trying to smother his exasperation at this traversing logic Carroll was following.

"I'm alone in the world. I can only depend on myself, and I have to be strong for everyone. It would be too hard to start over at this point in my life, and if I can keep doing this gig for at least ten more years, then I'll retire and fade away."

He reached over and gently lifted a stray curl off her cheek. "I cannot imagine Dr. Carroll Murphy ever fading away. Maybe getting the gray streaks in your hair covered or the crow's feet around your eyes touched up, but never any kind of fading operation."

Carroll giggled.

"I don't know what it is about you, but you can take me from the bottom of the barrel to being able to jump out to a soft landing in the blink of an eye." She stood and shook out the tartan, then gathered the pile of used tissues from the coffee table.

"I really need to be going now. It'll be hard enough to fly tomorrow with this nose all stuffed up and my eyes almost swollen shut."

"Can I call you after you return to California, Carroll?"

"Sure—yes, I'd really like that." She smiled broadly, wondering how her life could feel so changed in less than twenty-four hours.

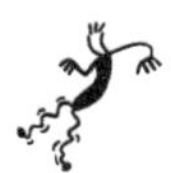

February 3, 2003

Southern California

Dr. Sutton greeted Carroll at his front door with the expected cup of herbal tea, and then he turned toward his office, clicking his cane with each step. Since his hip-replacement surgery the previous fall, he had struggled to get his gait back to normal. Carroll started to offer her arm to him, but she pulled back, knowing how stubbornly independent her mentor could be.

She seated herself in her usual place, and he waited for her to pull her client notes from her briefcase. When she continued to sit there, with no effort to retrieve the contents for their weekly discussions, he asked, "Well, are you going to tell me why you are grinning from ear to ear? You look like the cat that swallowed the canary."

"I met someone, Dr. S."

"Met someone? You? Isn't that a little out of character for you? What gives?" He smiled and tapped his pipe in the ashtray.

"I don't know. It certainly wasn't something I was looking for. I was having my usual solo vacation and enjoying it, thank you very much, when I skied upon an accident that had just happened. For some reason, I just completely froze on the spot, and probably would still be there on the slope if this really obnoxious guy hadn't come along and, quote, rescued me."

"Obnoxious guy? Would that be the same fellow who has turned your face into a virtual smile factory?"

Carroll giggled and blushed.

"I'm afraid so. Who would have believed it? He lives there—in Park City, I mean. And for the first time in a long time, I think I might be open to a relationship." She smiled, and her gaze disappeared into the fog that rolled onto the deck.

"Well, this is what I would call a true miracle, Carroll. Tell me more." Dr. Sutton's smile enveloped them both.

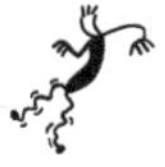

April 13, 2003

------Original message------

To: drcarroll@thesexladyonline.com

From: peggybsn@yahoo.com

Subject: Harleys

Dear Dr. Carroll:

Troy says he just has to have a Harley. And he says it has to be a Sportster because that is what Elvis rode. Now, you know I am not a risk-taker, but I just don't want to deny Troy the pleasure of having exactly the same experience as his hero had. Do you think Harleys are bad for people? I told Troy I will do what you tell me.

Thanks,

Peggy

P.S. Rainey has had a bad heart attack and it looks like she may not last much longer. Trixie is holding up pretty well, considering, but we all sure hope Rainey makes it past Mother's Day, for Trixie's sake.

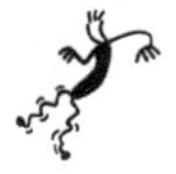

April 18, 2003

To: peggybsn@yahoo.com

From: drcarroll@thesexladyonline.com

Subject: Re: Harleys

Hi Peggy,

I don't know very much about about Harleys, so I think this is out of my league to be giving advice about. It seems to me you have always trusted Troy's judgment on cars and such. And I believe you said in addition to being a mechanic he has done a little auto racing also, so my guess is he understands the risk of such a vehicle. The only suggestion I would make is for him to sign up for a Harley riding class. A friend of mine says this is very important, no matter what skills a person already has.

Let me know what happens about Rainey.

Carroll

Carroll Murphy, PHD, CST, FAAST

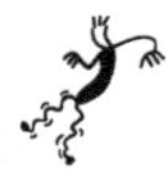

May 21, 2003

---------Original message---------

To: drcarroll@thesexladyonline.com

From: trixielovesvols@yahoo.com

Subject: Rainey's funeral

Dear Dr. Carroll:

Oh, Lord, honey, you just wouldn't believe what happened to Rainey at her memorial service. There we were in the New Hope Baptist Church, with Brother Fletcher greeting everybody just like it was a revival meeting, and Brother Spencer was getting ready to sing "Amazing Grace." And the next thing I knew, Rainey was flying to pieces. Well, I don't mean she was flying to pieces like when she was alive on this earth, but her ashes were flying all over the church.

Carroll was never surprised by anything she received from Trixie. Somehow, though, she had not expected to get a crisis-laden e-mail about Rainey's funeral. Prior to Rainey's death a couple of days ago, Trixie had posted regular updates, including the details of Rainey's last moments, and Carroll was impressed by the maturity Trixie was showing in the face of this loss.

After reading the first couple of lines of today's missive, Carroll backed away from the computer screen and unknotted the band around her flyaway red curls. She bent over and let her hair dangle through her knees and took a couple of deep yoga breaths.

This family is wearing me out, she sighed, setting her glasses on her desk while she rubbed the bridge of her nose, but as always, her fascination with Trixie's tales kept her returning to the saga.

Oh, Lord, I didn't know what Brother Fletcher was going to say when those Rainey bits started raining down—that's what Brother Fletcher said about it. He said, here we all were gathered for the memorial service to commemorate the life of Lorraine Brown Martin, who absolutely hated to miss a good party, and wouldn't you just know she would find a way to get herself there after all? And everybody agreed, and we heard more than a few "Amens" coming from the group in the second pew.

Well, honey, here's what happened. Little Walter Jr.—you remember he's my grandchild what was born from when Walter, my second boy, and that waitress hooked up for a while—well, little Walter Jr. had escaped from where his daddy was sitting in the family pew and had managed to crawl himself around behind the altar. Before anybody even saw him, he got his hands on that big urn where Rainey's ashes—the funeral home calls them "cremains"—were on view. I mean, after the service we were going to put them in the cemetery plot where all of six of us bought into—you know it's a whole lot cheaper these days to put everyone in one grave in little boxes than to dress everyone out in a highfalutin' casket. Anyway, little Walter Jr. is always trying to throw a football just like Peyton Manning does—you remember he was a Tennessee Vol before he turned Yankee and went to those Indianapolis Colts.

Carroll had no interest in the Tennessee Volunteers, but her disinterest had never stopped the Trollops from keeping her plied with bits of news about the Vol football team and its ups and downs. Never had Carroll encountered such fierce loyalty to a sports team or to a region of a country. She shook her head. *I think it borders on obsession.*

Well, even if little Walter Jr. is only four years old, he has been watching UT football since he was a little bitty baby, and anyway, I guess he thought that big old urn looked just like a football, and the next thing we knew, he had his hands on that glass football and his right arm cocked back just like Peyton, and he let loose a high, spiraling pass. But Lord, honey, none of his intended receivers could get there in time, and that urn flew about three feet through the air and came crashing down right in front of where Brother Spencer was smiling from ear to ear and singing "I once was lost but now I'm found."

And, honey, those ashes, well, they're not like the ashes what come from a fireplace. No sirree. They are more like little bits of gravel, and when they hit that marble floor in between the pulpit and the family pew, they bounced just like hailstones.

Carroll shook her head in disbelief. If she had not personally met Trixie and her cousin, Peggy, she would think somebody was making all this up, but her experience with these two women over the past six years convinced her that, without a trace of intent, these women and their families were about the most classic examples of dysfunction she had ever encountered.

Sighing again, Carroll pushed away from her computer screen and made herself a cup of herbal tea. At midnight, she could not afford to drink any more caffeine, although she would have preferred a bolder spot of black tea. She picked up her glasses and clicked the mouse, returning to Trixie's latest drama.

So, honey, that Brother Spencer, he just finished singing "Amazing Grace," and the congregation sat there not quite knowing what to do. Then Brother Fletcher walked up to the pulpit and said, "Families and neighbors, you have just witnessed a miracle. Lorraine Brown Martin—who all of you called Rainey—always told me she would be at her own funeral if she could find a way to get there, because she did not want anyone else to have the last word about her, and don't you just know, with the help of Jesus and her great-grandson, Rainey caused a hailstorm. If that don't constitute a modern-day miracle, then I don't know what does." Then he pounded the podium with his fist and launched into one of the fieriest sermons I have ever heard him preach and at the end, he offered an altar call to anyone who was not right with the Lord. And, honey, right there at Rainey's memorial service, when we were all singing "How Great Thou Art" with Troy just booming out on the refrain, three unsaved souls got right with Jesus.

Your friend,

Trixie

"No way. There is just no way this kind of thing happens!" shouted Carroll to her computer screen.

And somewhere in the depths of her soul, Carroll felt the familiar resonance she could not plumb.

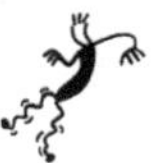

May 24, 2003

---------Original message---------

To: drcarroll@thesexladyonline.com

From: trixielovesvols@yahoo.com

Subject: Cancer

Dear Dr. Carroll:

Can a person get cancer from a cell phone?

E.R. told me there is a man in his church who had cancer of the ear where he always held his cell phone to talk, and then one night at prayer meeting, everybody put their hands on the man's head and prayed for God to take away the cancer, and wouldn't you know it, the next time they saw the man his cancer was all gone.

Your friend,

Trixie

P.S. Thank you so much for sending the flowers to Rainey's funeral. They were the prettiest ones there, and I showed them to every one of the Trollops when they came to pay their respects.

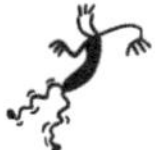

June 1, 2003

--------Original message-------

To: drcarroll@thesexladyonline.com

From: trixielovesvols@yahoo.com

Subject: Vacation

Dear Dr. Carroll:

Now I don't know what you can say that will help this mess, but I don't have anybody else to turn to with Rainey being gone, rest her soul. Here's what happened.

It was Memorial Day last week—well you probably already know that—anyway, me and Peggy and our kids and our kids' kids were going to get together and have a picnic. Now, it's not too much to expect of a family to get together once a year and cook out on that big old Weber grill Troy has in their backyard. After all, as I see it, the whole idea behind this holiday is to remember people in our past, and when Peggy and me get together, you can bet first one of us and then the other will pretty soon be talking about Rainey and Mama and how they must be up in Heaven just comparing notes about whose kin is doing better than the other, and honey, you can just bet which one of us comes out better.

Anyway, Troy started things off on the wrong foot. He and T. Roy were signed up to play in a three-day Memorial Day golf tournament and, as anybody knows, Memorial Day is always on a Monday, which meant they'd been playing golf on Sunday. Now E.R. thinks it's a sin to play golf on Sunday—he says the only thing any God-fearing person ought to do on the Lord's Day is go to church, read the Bible, and eat lunch at the cafeteria.

Now, between you and me, I don't know what he expects those cafeteria workers to do about going to church and reading the Bible if they spend the whole day cooking and serving food to people like him, but he says there are some people who get excused and they are those people. It just don't make sense to me the way he works things out, but he has strict lists in his head of "rights" and "wrongs," and nobody is going to change his mind.

Well, honey, it never had exactly been a secret, but when E.R. got wind that Troy and T. Roy and Troy's best friend, Wayne, had headed off on Sunday morning to play golf, he went into one of those preaching fits (that's what I call them) of his, and he told me there was no way he was going to go to any barbecue with any heathen, and that was that.

So, I said to him I would just go by myself anyway, since Calvin and Bruce could come by and pick me up, and then E.R. just about lost it. He said, and I am quoting him so I hope I don't offend you, "The very idea of that fag son of yours and his corn-holer boyfriend coming by this house just about makes me puke," and he said I had better make up my mind right now which it would be—him or my "sweet ass boy."

Dr. Carroll, I have never been so upset in just about my whole life. I mean, Calvin has never been anything but kind to me and to E.R. and, yes, I would rather my oldest son liked girls better than boys, but he had every opportunity to like girls and never showed one inkling of liking them. Now, I don't exactly know whether being gay is biology or something somebody chooses, but in Calvin's case, he has been like this his whole life, and I don't think anybody or anything will change him. It's not like he is out running around or anything. Once he met Bruce, they have been a twosome, and they seem just like two peas in a pod.

Well anyway, honey, E.R. stayed home and pouted, and I got my deviled eggs and potato salad all together and just rode over to Peggy's as big as Pete with Calvin and Bruce. And, honey, you know I have told you on more than one occasion that Troy doesn't much like the idea of two men being lovers either, but at least he has some manners, and you would never have known anything about the way he feels from the way he treated those boys. Now if you can believe this, Troy and Bruce actually get along pretty well, now that he's found out Bruce plays golf, too. I even heard him say if Bruce really does have a six handicap, then he will play a round with him any day. Now I don't know what being handicapped has to do with it, but maybe Troy thought he might be more handicapped than Bruce, 'cause he looked around at T. Roy and said point blank, "Son, you get my back and if Bruce even comes close to grabbing my butt when I bend over to mark my ball, then it is all over," and T. Roy just winked back at his dad.

Frankly, Dr. Carroll, I don't think Bruce or Calvin or any other gay guy would try to rub Troy's butt cheeks, as big as they are. I sometimes don't even see how Peggy can get worked up enough to make love with him, but then I guess love is blind.

But here's the point I am writing about tonight. E.R. told me when I came home from the picnic that our summer vacation plans are off, after what happened this weekend. I said, "Why E.R., you have been looking forward to going to Holy Land USA for the last five years, ever since you read about it in the *Enquirer.* What in the world has got into you to change your plans?"

Honey, that man has not talked about one other single thing for more than a year, since he found out he could get two whole weeks off together because of his seniority, and he could rent an R.V. and drive it down to Florida. Now to tell you the truth, I haven't been all that excited about the Holy Land Park. Really, I would rather go to Disney World, but he says he won't set foot inside their gates because they sponsor "gay days," so I guess being practically next door is almost the real thing. And he told me we could even take a little detour and stop off in North Carolina and visit the world's largest Ten Commandments, which would truly be a sight to see.

Ever since I saw the movie about those Ten Commandments when I was in high school, I have wanted to see the real things, and there they are, just one state away from us, with the words in concrete block letters five feet high! E.R. even showed me a picture from the *Enquirer,* and it said the Roman numerals are ten feet high.

Well, it is also supposed to be my vacation and Lord, knows I do need one after all I have been through with Rainey dying and everything. If E.R. doesn't go, then I will just have to sit in this doublewide and look at him and I think we will both lose our minds over that. So, Dr. Carroll, what do you think I should do?

Your friend,

Trixie

P.S. Thanks for asking how I am doing. It has just about tore me up to let go of Rainey, but I guess I don't have much choice.

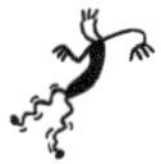

June 3, 2003

To: trixielovesvols@yahoo.com

From: drcarroll@thesexladyonline.com

Subject: Re: Vacation

Trixie—Sorry E.R. is giving you fits. Why don't you and Peggy and some girlfriends get together and take a trip on your own? You deserve it! Please send me a postcard from wherever you go. And send one to E.R. too!

Carroll

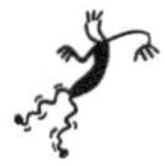

June 20, 2003

To: drcarroll@thesexladyonline.com

From: trixielovesvols@yahoo.com

Subject: Re: Re: Vacation

Dear Dr. Carroll:

Thanks! Hope you got my postcard from L.A. All of us girls and my little Strudel just piled into Peggy's SUV—she'd just finished her semester in school, and girl, was she ever ready for some fun time—and we started down that road, and before you even knew it, there we were on that beach, and we sure did have us a good old time. I don't think E.R. even hardly knew I was gone, and that just suits me fine.

Frankly, Dr. Carroll, I am about ready to give up men in general. I just am worn out with having men try to tell me what I can and cannot do. Thank God, E.R. is not interested in having sex with anybody, as far as I can tell, because if he did want to do it with me, I just don't think I could find the spirit to do it. The last straw came when E.R. told me last week after Strudel and I came home, I had to choose between his two legs and my dog's four legs, because there was not room in his house for both.

Well, I declare, it was no choice at all for me. I'll take four legs and a wet tongue any day over two legs and a sharp tongue. So I just said, 'Excuse me for living, but I think I will just take my little bitty baby dog and find myself another place to live, thank you very much.' I don't know how we will make it on my pay from the salon, but I would rather starve and be under my own roof than to be kept by a man who is going to try to control me.

Your friend,

Trixie

P.S. I hope you know which L.A. I mean.

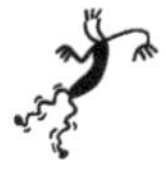

June 30, 2003

Southern California

"Dr. S., since Trixie's mother died she has about run me crazy with her e-mails. There is some kind of crisis going on every day in the woman's life."

"Carroll, why don't you tell her to get herself a real therapist—you are resigning from that job?"

"I know, I know. But somehow I just keep getting hooked back in. I'll think it over. See you next week."

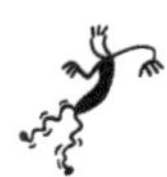

PART FIVE: RECONCILIATION and DANCING

July 2003

When Mitch first mentioned to Carroll he was a golfer and she might enjoy playing, she was less than enthusiastic about the suggestion. As a small child, her dad took her along with him to the golf range, where he hit balls with amazing accuracy despite having only one leg. At the time, Carroll took it for granted all dads could hit golf balls, and she never once questioned his constant efforts to keep balance on one leg while at the same time swinging a golf club almost 380 degrees. Only later, when she had a client who was an arm amputee and played golf in the Amputee Golf Association tour, did she begin to appreciate her father's innate athleticism.

Mitch had his heart set on playing Torrey Pines. With Carroll living a little more than an hour's drive from the most famous public course in southern California, going there was a no-brainer for him. It was easy for him to get away for a long weekend whenever he chose, since he did not have office hours on Fridays. Knowing he was coming to visit had been the impetus for Carroll to sign up for a series of beginner lessons with one of the best-known golf instructors in the country. Petra LeBlanc's School of Golf regularly made the Top 100 list in *Women's Golf Digest,* and Carroll was not disappointed. After the end of the six half-day lessons, Carroll felt comfortable enough to join Mitch for a practice round at a local public course before he took on the site of the annual Buick Open.

“I think you have real potential, Carroll,” encouraged Mitch, as they walked back to his rental car. “You are very competitive and you have a great touch around the greens. I think with a little practice you could have a game.”

“Maybe,” Carroll grudgingly allowed, “but I don’t think I could ever be good enough to play regularly.”

“That’s why golf has a handicap system. Granted, you’re not ever going to play with the likes of Annika—and I’m not ever going to play with Tiger—but it doesn’t mean we can’t go out and have a game.”

It was hard to argue with Mitch, who always was so positive toward her.

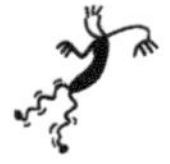

August 14, 2003

---------Original message---------

To: drcarroll@thesexladyonline.com

From: trixielovesvols@yahoo.com

Subject: Cancer

Dear Dr. Carroll:

Do you think I will get cancer from having my hair dyed for so long? There was an article in the *Enquirer* about some lady in Washington state who got head cancer after she kept her hair blonde for so many years, and E.R. circled it in red and told me to read it. Lord, honey, you know that man has been on me for years to let my natural hair grow out, but if I did, I am afraid the sight of those roots would be enough to scare away half the people who come into that salon where I work. But I sure don't want to get cancer of the scalp or any such thing as that.

Your friend,

Trixie

P.S. I did not move out yet, but I am still thinking about it. He makes me so mad.

P.S.S. I told him I would let Strudel sleep with me any old time I wanted to and he just better not try to stop me!

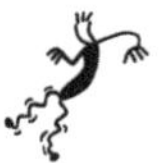

August 18, 2003

To: trixielovesvols@yahoo.com

From: drcarroll@thesexladyonline.com

Subject: Re: Cancer

Trixie—I don't know much about cancer, so I would suggest you ask your primary care provider about those risks.

Carroll

P.S. I am glad you are holding your ground with E.R.

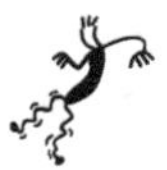

September 1, 2003

--------Original message--------

To: drcarroll@thesexladyonline.com

From: trixielovesvols@yahoo.com

Subject: More Trollops

Dear Dr. Carroll:

Guess what? Crystal has a sister by the name of Astrid who lives in Peoria, Illinois, and when Crystal told Astrid about the Trollops, why Astrid just said on the spot she knew six more girls who qualified, and don't you just know, now there is another chapter and they call themselves the Flamingo Girls because they always wear stuff that has flamingos on it.

Your friend,

Trixie

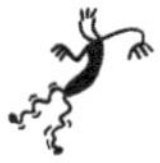

September 13, 2003

The message light was blinking when Carroll entered her condo, and she immediately checked her caller ID. Ever since her Uncle Morton had tracked down her home number and left the message about her mother's emergency surgery last year, she had had her guard up. She had considered changing the number, which was already unlisted, but for various reasons she had decided to leave it the same.

"Hey, Carroll, guess what? I am a free woman! Pete signed over everything to me, and I have more money than I know what to do with! So I am going to start spending it as fast as I can, and the first place I am spending it is to come see you."

Janie Hoffman had not visited Carroll in Los Angeles since Carroll's wedding to Brian in 1968, when Janie had been pregnant with Nathan. The two friends had managed to do lunch or dinner a few times when Carroll had been in the Chicago area, but once Pete's company transferred him to

Charlotte in 1999, they almost never could manage to coordinate their schedules for a visit.

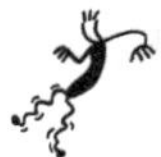

Sitting in Carroll's favorite neighborhood Italian restaurant a week later, Janie ordered a glass of red wine and Carroll asked for sparkling water with lime.

"What gives?" Janie asked.

"Oh, I think that wine sometimes gives me a headache. Sometimes I just lay off it."

"Well, thank goodness that has not happened to me. I could not get through dinner without a great bottle of cab. There is one good thing I will say about old Pete—he loved his wine, and he had a ton of it in his cellar. When that judge told him he had to split the wine cellar with me, I thought he was going to pass out right there in the courtroom! And you should see the cellar I put in my new house." She whistled for emphasis, just as the waitperson arrived with their entrees.

"I know you said in your holiday note last year that things were rocky between you and Pete, but this seems awfully sudden. What happened?" asked Carroll.

"Pete—if ever a person were aptly named it is him—Pete the Pecker—that's what all my golfing buddies call him," she grinned and winked, then continued.

"I swear, when I found out the real reason he got transferred to Charlotte was because he was screwing one of the junior partners in the Lake Forest office, I said to myself 'those first wives got it right—don't get mad, get even.' And if I do say so myself, I more than got even."

She raised her wine glass to clink with Carroll's water, and they nodded in harmony, smiling into each other's eyes.

"Why did you decide to move back to Chicago?" Carroll asked between bites of her whole grain fettuccine.

"Well, for one thing, I missed my girls' golf group. We played together every Tuesday for twenty-five years, and some of us would also get together on Wednesdays at the club and play mah-jongg and they don't do much of that—mah-jongg, I mean—in Charlotte. Also, you know, my mom is getting pretty frail these days, and I thought since I was going to get a new house anyway close to our old neighborhood, I would just add on a suite for her, and then I could look in on her whenever she needs me. Of course, we have round-the-clock help for her, but sometimes a mother just needs a daughter around."

Janie searched Carroll's face for some emotion, then seeing none she continued.

"I ran into *your* mother at the market last week and she asked me about you. She looked pretty well, but she is very thin. I didn't tell her I was coming to see you."

Carroll put down her fork and spoon and patted the corner of her white cotton napkin to her mouth. She took a drink of ice water, feeling the cold liquid wash down her pasta, then she breathed slowly and deliberately from her gut. Fixing her gaze steadily on her friend's face, she locked their eyes in place, then cleared her throat before speaking.

"Janie, we've been friends for a long time, so please don't take this the wrong way, but if you ever again mention my mother to me, I will not see you anymore. Please, for my sake, let bygones be bygones."

Janie hesitated, her forked bite of grilled salmon suspended in midair. Her face began to burn, and tears welled in her eyes.

"Okay, okay, I hear you. But I guess I just don't see how you can keep up such a barrier against the only person in the world who is your flesh and blood. I know for sure in my family, if we're not all talking to each other at least once a week, my mother is going nuts. But I agree to stick with your rules. I will say this, though, if you ever want to tell me what it was that finally came between the two of you, I am open to hearing it."

"I can assure you that will never happen in my lifetime, Janie. It's done, and I don't choose to look back. Now, can we talk about you and your children and grandchildren?"

Carroll twirled her fettuccine against the spoon and smoothed a little Alfredo sauce on it before lifting it to her mouth. The ritual did only a little to soothe her aching spirit.

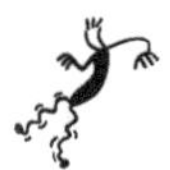

September 22, 2003

Southern California

"Dr. S., I had a nasty run-in with Janie when she was here last week. She was pushing me to make contact with my mother, and I simply refuse to do so."

"Tell me more about you and your mother, Carroll," he invited.

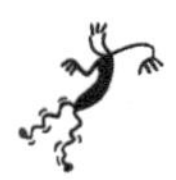

October 28, 1963

Carroll had just left her last class of the day—Western Civ—when she picked up her mother's weekly letter from her campus mailbox in the student center and walked outside in the cool of the late fall afternoon, looking for a bench where she could sit and read uninterrupted. Except for an occasional brief note from Janie who was at Colorado State and a monthly notice from the U.S. government confirming her Social Security dependent benefit payment had been deposited into her checking account, she rarely had other personal mail. After six weeks of college, she was feeling disillusioned.

"Frankly," she told Melinda, "except for Western Civ, all my classes are just repetitions of what I did in high school. I think I made a big mistake by not going to Northwestern back home. I just don't think I am cut out for this kind of college."

Earlier that afternoon, the Western Civ class giggled nervously when Dr. Barkley, their newly minted instructor, told them, "A year ago today, I was getting ready to defend my dissertation on Communism in the Western Hemisphere. If Khrushchev had not backed down and ordered the missiles out of Cuba, neither you nor I would probably have been here in class this afternoon reviewing Western Civilization."

It seemed to Carroll that it had been a long year.

She sat on a bench near a giant magnolia tree in the shadow of Monmouth Hall, holding the unopened letter from her mother.

This had better not be another of her poor me letters, Carroll thought, as she lifted the back flap and started to pull the letter out of the envelope. *For once, I wish she could think of me and not just about herself and how sad and lonely she is. For God's sake, I will be seventeen tomorrow, and I have a life I would like to lead myself!*

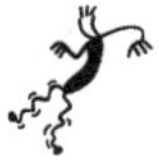

October 22, 1963

Dearest Carroll,

It feels like there are a million miles between us, rather than the 489 actual miles. I know you need to act strong, but sometimes I long to have you crawl into my lap and let me hold you, as I did when you were so small. Everything has changed for us in the past ten years since your daddy has been gone. I have tried to do what I thought was needed to help you have the most normal life I could provide, but I know I have failed in some areas.

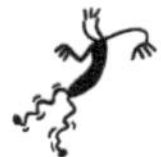

You bet you've failed. A tear fell onto her white blouse, hitting the circle pin which she had carefully attached to the oxford-cloth collar earlier today. She hated wearing this garb, but without it she felt she looked even more peculiar to these young women, so she had splurged on two outfits of the Warfield standard attire during rush, and now she felt obligated to wear them. As the dab of moisture rolled over the chrome finish onto her madras plaid skirt, she was startled to realize someone was standing in front of her.

"May I be of assistance, Miss—uh-uh—I'm sorry, but I cannot recall your name. I know you sit in the front row of my class, but at this point in the semester, I don't have everyone's names committed to memory."

Carroll steepled her fingers over her eyes to shield them from the low-hanging fall sun. It took a moment for the shape of the tall figure to confirm his identity. The outline of his head moved across the sun's path, allowing Carroll to more clearly see her professor's face, with his thin lips and aquiline nose. The sun spots in front of her eyes receded, and Robert Barkley's corduroy jacket resumed its caramel color. By most standards, he was not a handsome man, but to the several hundred freshmen women who took his Western Civ class, he was mesmerizing. His distinct voice, with just a grace note of a southern drawl, spoke again.

"Miss Murphy, I believe it is?"

His lean body and the unlit pipe held in the palm of his right hand were the two things she would always remember about Professor Robert Barkley. Those and his impeccable manners.

"No, thanks. I'm fine," Carroll muttered, her hoarse, wet voice coming out with more the texture of a cough than of a sentence.

"Well, Miss, you don't look or sound fine. Could we have a cup of coffee and you could tell me what has happened?"

"I don't think so. I have to be somewhere," Carroll lied. "Good-bye."

She ran for the dorm, where she could hide her shame at letting her feelings be so public. It was not Art's way, and she could feel her father's eyes on her blotched face, while Dr. Barkley's gaze penetrated her back.

You must be strong, pal. Never look back. Always keep your eyes glued to where you are going.

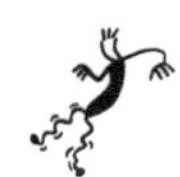

Carroll heard the news as she was on her way to her afternoon biology lab. That class, along with almost everything else on the Warfield campus, was canceled as all eyes became glued to the black-and-white TV sets that had been set up in strategic locations. Both students and faculty had congregated wherever there was a TV to try to make some sense of the story coming out of Dallas.

She guessed Robert Barkley had been standing behind her for some time, when she turned and faced him.

"How about that cup of coffee now, Miss Murphy?" he invited. She was glad to join him in doing something normal on a day when the world seemed to have been turned upside down.

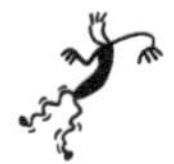

When classes resumed on Monday afternoon after the state funeral, she sat in her front-row seat, soaking up Dr. Barkley's every word about the effect of the assassination and the subsequent transfer of power on the stability of the world.

"This event, while tragic, is a great example of the near-perfection of the U.S. Constitution," he taught, pointing out the contrasts between the United States and other countries when such sudden disruptions took place.

Carroll felt her face redden when his eyes swept over her, and she scribbled furiously in her spiral notebook. When class ended she hung back, waiting to see if he would ask her to coffee again. She was not disappointed.

Thanksgiving break started at midday on Wednesday, so Carroll hurriedly stopped by Dr. Barkley's office to tell him good-bye, but he was already gone. She left him a brief note to thank him for comforting her during the five grief-laden days, adding her mother's home phone number at the bottom of the note, and then she headed to the depot with another coed who had hired a cab.

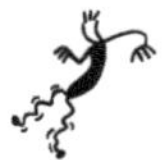

Carroll hesitated before stepping off the train into the cavernous belly of Chicago's Union Station. *What kind of shape will she be in?* Carroll wondered.

Frances waved and Carroll signaled back, pushing a curl back out of her eyes. It was unusually cold for this early in winter in Chicago, and she had already buttoned up her jacket and pulled her knee socks up as far as possible under the pleated wool skirt that came down well over her knees, as required by the dress code at the university. *It's crazy we can't wear slacks in public!* she silently ranted, remembering how the orientation committee had told the new freshmen class that such dress was unladylike.

"That rule's not long for this world," Carroll had whispered to the coed sitting next to her.

Do I look any different? She had always been thin—maybe even too thin for her almost five-foot-eight frame, but after snacking on chocolate-chip cookies and other goodies in the dorm, she knew she and many of her classmates were on their way to the famed freshman fifteen.

She probably won't ask me any questions. The only thing that matters to her is her next drink, or whether my socks match. "You only get one chance to make a good first impression," Frances had preached on an almost daily basis.

She once had asked her mother why she had never dated after Art's death, but Frances had just said there was no room in her heart for anyone but Art, and eventually her friends stopped asking her to be a fourth at the bridge table when they had an extra man around.

Carroll's face came closer to her mother's through the mass of people moving in and out of the train platforms. Unconsciously, she pulled out a small pocket mirror and checked her hair. *She'll look me up and down,* she thought, her jaw clenching. *I'll just pretend everything's fine like I've done hundreds of times before.*

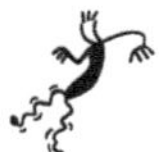

It felt good to sleep in late on Thanksgiving morning. Frances had worked the graveyard shift at the hospital and wouldn't be up until the afternoon, so Carroll could eat a leisurely breakfast and watch the Macy's parade on TV, a welcome respite from the national mourning. She and Frances were going to have Thanksgiving dinner that night with the Rubens, but her mother had told her Janie wouldn't be there, since it was so far from Colorado and such a short span of time to make the trip.

Nothing's changed on her end, she thought, seeing her mother's breakfast plate and utensils stacked in the sink. Carroll washed them and put them in the drainer on the counter with her own clean ones.

She was startled when the phone rang, and she lifted the receiver on the first ring.

"Is it really you? You are here?" squealed Carroll into the phone. "How did your folks manage to get you all the way home for Thanksgiving? . . .They splurged for an airplane ticket? . . . Oh, Janie, you are so lucky to have the parents you have." Carroll was sincere. She never held it against any of her friends when their parents were there for them. "I'll be right over. Don't move. I have so much to tell you!"

Carroll crept into her mother's bedroom to get the car keys from her purse. She started the car and quietly backed it out the driveway into the alley, and then turned north towards Janie's house, marveling at how the old neighborhood had hardly changed in the two months she had been away.

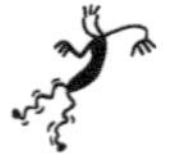

"There you have it, Dr. S. When I got to Janie's, she was so wrapped up in her wonderful new world at Colorado State she didn't have the time or interest to hear how awful my college life was, so I just stopped trying to tell her. I hung out at her house again during Christmas break after the blow-up with my mother, but she was mooning all over the place about her new boyfriend, Pete, so I didn't really see how she could listen to my troubles. Their house was just as full of people coming and going as if they were celebrating the Christmas holiday and, well, I just kind of got lost in the shuffle like the proverbial redheaded stepchild."

She smoothed her hair and grinned at hearing her unplanned metaphor, then continued more seriously. "Then, after I withdrew from Warfield and moved to Oregon, I hardly ever talked to Janie any more until Brian and I were getting married, and by then she was married and having babies. After that, we just mostly went our separate ways."

Dr. Sutton leaned back in his desk chair and pulled on the pipe stem in his mouth.

"So are you holding it against Janie after all these years that she wasn't there for you?"

"Not holding it against her, but I guess I wonder what she could really understand, since our paths have gone in such different directions. And I simply do not trust that my mother, who I just found out is still alive and still trying to snare me, won't wheedle information out of Janie."

"Carroll, why do you fight so hard against giving your mother another chance? It's been forty years since you walked out of her life. That's a lot of water over the dam, for God's sake." He stopped, but Carroll did not reply. "You are a big proponent of forgiveness—you tell your clients they don't necessarily have to reconcile with the person they are estranged from, but they need to . . . uhh," he flipped through his notes. "Let's see, several sessions ago you were quoting that forgiveness book you really like, and you said, 'Sometimes it's hardest to forgive the one you most need to forgive, especially if what you need to forgive is they were not who you wanted them to be.'"

Carroll glared at her supervisor and bit her lip.

He continued, "Your mother was a human being. She made mistakes. I know you thought at the time she should have been above using alcohol to comfort herself, but she probably had an illness. She wasn't a bad person. Just sick."

"You have no idea what she did to me, Dr. S." Carroll's eyes narrowed and the tears welled up.

"Well, that's true, since you won't tell me the full story. Have you ever considered how you'll feel if this doesn't get resolved before she dies?"

"I never give it any thought, thank you very much." Carroll reached for her briefcase and walked out of his office. She took a deep breath and held it until she reached her car.

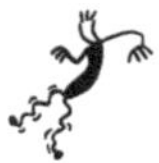

October, 2003

--------Original message---------

To: drcarroll@thesexladyonline.com

From: trixielovesvols@yahoo.com

Subject: Golf and G-spots

Dear Dr. Carroll,

Peggy will not write to you about this, so I decided to do it for her. Now I know you keep telling us we should just speak up for ourselves, but, honey, sometimes I think Peggy just has too much medical brains and not enough living brains, and she says she does not want to bother you about this one. But Lord, honey, if we can't ask you about such things, then who can we ask?

Here's the deal. Now you know Troy and Peggy have been together almost every minute of their lives, except for when Troy is working on those cars or playing golf, or when Peggy is working or studying, and that is a lot of time to spend together, so I can see how they might get a little tired of doing the same things over and over in the bedroom, if you get my drift. And, honey, I do remember what ole Father Bob, bless his heart, said at that wedding in Northern Virginia. Even if he was a little too friendly from all the wine and then got that glint in his eye for me, the man did make some good points, and I will give him credit for that. Anyway, here's what happened.

Troy had come in from one of his golf games—that man will play golf outside, even if it is snowing up to the bejeebies—and he decided to tell Peggy a joke he had heard from one of his buddies on the course. It seems Wayne asked the group if they knew the difference between a golf ball and the G-spot, and right away Roger said, "Sure, I'd look for my golf ball for as long as it takes to find it!" And Troy just thought that was the funniest thing he had ever heard. He could not for the life of himself figure out why Peggy got so huffy after he told her this.

Now, honey, Peggy does not get very touchy about most things. She is one of the most even-tempered and sweet people I have ever known, but every little bit, when Troy has been playing just a little too much golf and has been neglecting his husbandry duties, so to speak, then that girl will let herself get worked into a little tiny pout. I mean, a few years ago Troy had been playing so much golf she had hardly seen him for over three months, except to find his dirty socks under the bed or his golf shorts needing a new pocket from where he had been stuffing them full of those old tees, or whatever the heck it is men put in their pockets when they are playing golf. Well, anyway, Troy came home one Saturday afternoon and noticed Peggy was acting a little miffed, so he thought he had missed their anniversary again.

Now that boy can remember just about every golf score he has ever had and can tell you exactly what happened on each hole, no matter what course he has been on, but for the life of him, he cannot remember when their wedding anniversary is. Now since their anniversary is always the week before Valentine's Day, you'd think he could get those two dates linked together each year, but, bless his heart, he just cannot keep it straight. Sometimes he will call me up and say, "Hey, Trix, you gotta help me out. I think I've done missed Valentine's again this year." And I will say back to him, "Troy, dadgummit, Valentine's Day is always on February 14 and your anniversary is February 10, so why can't you just learn that?" Anyway, it does not ever seem to stick with him.

So anyway, he was feeling real guilty, so he hightailed it to Victoria's Secret and bought Peggy the tiniest little negligee you have ever seen. I mean, after all, she is a grown woman, and even when she was a teenager I don't think she wore a size two, but here Troy was buying her a size two red nightie, and he brought it in as proud as a peacock and handed it to her. She took one look at it and turned right around and walked off and did not even say "how do you do?" and the next thing Troy saw of it was when he went to bed that night and laying there right next to his pillow on the bed was his golf bag and the red negligee was draped over it and Peggy had written him a note. "Dear Troy, I hope you get hours of pleasure with this old bag and this size two whatever it is, 'cause you sure are not going to get any pleasure with me for a while."

And that Troy just about dropped his tail between his legs, because he knew he was for sure cut off, and he had better find a way to get back in Peggy's good graces. And he did. Get back in her good graces, I mean. Now she did not tell me exactly what had happened between them, but I know she eventually forgave him, and they kissed and made up, so to speak, and I think their sex life must have improved because he seemed a lot calmer, and she usually had a big smile on her face.

So, anyway, when he told her that golf ball joke, I think he stepped on a new little minefield, so to speak. Peggy started crying, and she didn't quit crying for most of two days. She called me up and came over here—it was a Sunday night and E.R. was at his church, like he always is on Sunday night, so I made us some margaritas and just kept telling Peggy whatever it was it was going to be okay. Honey, honest and truly, I did not know what I was supposed to do, but then I thought to myself, "What would Dr. Carroll do in this situation?" so I just up and invented you inside me, and if I do say so myself, I think I have some talent for this counseling business. Now I don't want you to think I am about to come out there to California and take over your job. No sirree! That would not be my cup of tea. But when my cousin needs my help, then I can certainly step right up, thank you very much.

So here's what she said. She said Troy and herself had been working on his being a more active sex partner in their relationship. Now, it seems getting on towards their sixties—and remember, Troy is already there, because he is two years older than Peggy—well, anyway, things had changed somewhat for them in bed, so to speak, because of their age. Now, I wouldn't really know much about that personally, you'll remember, because E.R.

and me—well, we don't have sex, so I am like a born-again virgin, I guess, after not having sex for over seven years. But I tried to listen just as best as I could, and when Peggy told me she had needed Troy to be more "hands on" in their sex life, it did make sense to me. Lord knows, a lot of what used to come naturally to me when I was younger needs a lot of help these days, so I guess it's true in sex, also.

It seems they had been working on his finding her G-spot because on the few occasions when he had found it or had been close to it, she had really been stirred up in ways she had not really felt for years, so she was pretty much liking what he was learning to do. Then he comes in from golf and all but tells her that finding a G-spot is not nearly as important as finding a golf ball, and honey, I can see exactly why her feelings were so badly hurt. Why, that is just a terrible thing to tell someone! And I almost got up right there and went to call up Troy and tell him what I thought, but then I remembered what that other lady who writes in the newspaper says—to MYOB—so I just sat there and said, "Oh, yes. I can see why what he said would bother you. Tell me more." I heard you on Oprah not long ago going over those things for people to say when someone is melting down, so I said to myself, "I can just be Dr. Carroll right here in my living room," and do you know, it really worked! After a while, Peggy quit crying, and she went to the bathroom and fluffed herself up and honey, I didn't even have to tell her what to do next. She said she would work it out on her own! What do you think about that?

Your friend,

Trixie

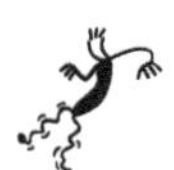

November 20, 2003

To: trixielovesvols@yahoo.com

From: drcarroll@thesexladyonline.com

Subject: Re: Golf and G-spots

Trix—You're doing great! Want to come work for me?

Carroll

P.S. Hope things are still going better with E.R.

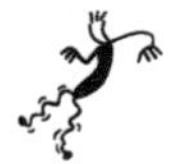

December 6, 2003

---------Original message---------

To: drcarroll@thesexladyonline.com

From: jrsfreeagain@aol.com

Subject: Us

C— Great seeing you in L.A.! Note my new e-mail address—no more Hoffman for me—back to my Rubens roots!

Wish you could have been with us for Thanksgiving, just like the old days. Can you believe they're selling Marshall Field's again? This time it's May Company who's the buyer, but I'll bet Macy's will eventually buy *them* out. And when that happens, I'll bet they won't even keep the name. Remember how much fun we used to have going into downtown Chicago on the El with your Aunt Ann to eat at the Walnut Room? You would have thought we were really something doing that tearoom stuff. Remember Mrs. Herring's chicken pot pie? Yum! I miss those fun times we used to have.

Bye. Love you.

J

P.S. Let me know when you're coming to Chicago next. I don't want to just have to catch my oldest friend on Oprah. Want to show you around a little where I live. I'm so excited you're a golfer now. Maybe we could get in eighteen holes in the spring sometime when you're coming in for a taping. I have an extra set of clubs you can use.

P.S. again. I wanted to clue you in—I've quit sending holiday letters—feels wonderful to be a free woman!

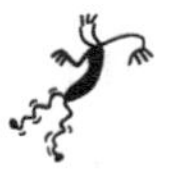

December 11, 2003

To: jrsfreeagain@aol com

From: drcarroll@thesexladyonline.com

Subject: Re: Us

Hi Janie—Glad to hear from you, and so glad we could get together when you were here. Yes, I remember the fun we had at Marshall Field's. I haven't had pot pie that good in almost forty years. I will definitely let you know when I'm coming into town, but sometimes I don't have much free time when I'm taping a show. It gets a little harried trying to keep everything together. Thank goodness for Barbara in my office who manages everything so well for me.

Carroll

P.S. Oh, by the way, I broke 100 for the first time last week!

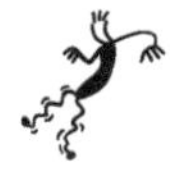

December 15, 2003

Southern California

"You seem very quiet today, Carroll. Want to tell me what's going on?"

"Oh, just thinking, I guess, Dr. S."

"About...?"

"Well, Mitch wants me to spend the week after Christmas with him in Sonoma. I don't know whether I'm up for that."

"Why not? That seems like a good thing from where I sit. You seem to really care for him, and from what you've told me, he puts no pressure on you to be or do anything."

Carroll smiled and accepted the fresh cup of tea he offered. She stood to walk to the patio door, glad today for the clearing of the early fog so she could see out to the waves.

"I don't know, Dr. S. On the one hand, I do welcome having Mitch in my life, but on the other hand, I've kept myself apart from a relationship for such a long time that I'm not sure I'd know what to do. It's funny—you know, of course, that I spend every day giving advice about such things to my clients and I do the same on the show, but when it comes to taking my own advice, I'm about a failure."

She sipped slowly, walking back to her chair. Dr. Sutton chewed on his pipe stem, his eyes twinkling.

"You're afraid you'll lose him, aren't you, like what happened with your dad and with Brian."

"Yeah, I guess so, but it's hard for me to admit that. I learned so many years ago to keep myself buttoned up, and it's just not all that easy to unbutton, so to speak."

"Well, he doesn't seem to be pushing you to physically unbutton, so maybe we could talk about the possibility of you emotionally opening up a little."

"Dr. S., sometimes talking to you is about as much fun as having a root canal."

She grinned and sipped her tea, shivering despite its warmth.

"Here, wrap this throw around your shoulders. I love the breeze as it comes through the open door but I don't want you freezing sitting here."

"I don't think it's the breeze making me shiver, Dr. S."

He chewed quietly, never taking his kind eyes off his protégé.

"I'm a fraud, Dr. S. A living, breathing fraud," Carroll said quietly.

"A fraud?"

"Yes, I know lots of therapists say the thought of not really being who they seem to be haunts them in the background, but in my case, it's really true."

"How so?"

"Well, for one, I'm not really the world's most compassionate therapist. I have learned to act like someone who cares deeply, but the truth is that lots of times I'm saying to myself, 'Why don't they just get over this and move on. Why do they have to keep ruminating over the same thing for years?'"

"In other words, Carroll, why don't they become like you, since nothing in your past affects you?"

Carroll bit her lip fiercely and hung her head. *Don't look back!* she heard her dad say. *We have to be strong!* her mother echoed.

Minutes passed and Dr. Sutton sat quietly, chewing his pipe stem. He reached over to the crystal ashtray on the table next to his desk and tapped the imaginary ashes into the bowl.

"Want to try telling me what's going on in your head?" he invited.

"Oh, I was just thinking about a woman with whom I've just started working—we'll call her Blanche. She came to see me because she's been married for three years, and she and her husband have not yet consummated their marriage."

"Oh?"

"I know that seems hard to believe in this day and age, especially in California, but when we started to look under the surface, it actually made a lot of sense—at least it did to me. Seems she had had an affair with a married man when she was in her early twenties. She got pregnant and because of her religion she didn't think she should have an abortion, so she moved to another state and gave birth, and then she gave up the baby for adoption. That was ten years ago, and she says she can't put what she did—giving up the baby—out of her mind."

"So, you're saying the earlier experience unconsciously blocks her intimacy with her husband?

"As far as I can tell it does. I keep telling her that she made the right decision at the time, and her child probably has been way better off being with parents who have means, rather than having lived with a single mom."

"And...?"

"And she agrees, but she still can't seem to put it behind her."

"So what does this bring up in you, Carroll?'

"Well, of course I think about how my life would have been different if I hadn't miscarried after Brian died. How I would have been a single parent myself, but somehow I just can't seem to connect with her emotions on this. I mean, I've certainly never been promiscuous, but I've also not been inhibited about having sex on occasion when the opportunity was right."

"Well, when we last talked, you volunteered that you and Mitch have not yet had intercourse and you've been seeing each other for, what, going on eight months? So it sounds a little like you and Blanche have something in common."

"That's true. The thing is, I'm open to being sexual with him, but he just keeps saying not to rush things. That when the time is right it will happen. Frankly, Dr. S., I think he may be intimidated by what I do for a living and he keeps procrastinating, afraid he won't be able to perform."

"Could be" Dr. Sutton answered, *but if I were a betting person, I'd say he knows exactly what he's doing, and by letting Carroll be in charge, he's giving her time to seek him out. Smart man!*

"So it's difficult for me to put myself in her shoes and, frankly, I have a hard time feeling empathy for her. It's in her past, and both she and the child are better off at this point than if she had made another decision."

She shifted in her chair.

"So for you, it's just better to keep moving forward and to be stoic?"

Carroll bit her lip and stanched the tears that were brimming.

"Is there something else?" Dr. Sutton leaned forward a little, and Carroll looked over at him, receiving his warm smile into her heart.

"Well, she says she feels like somebody tattooed a big scarlet A across her chest, and she has to say no with her body in order to atone. It makes no sense to me. She made a mistake—used bad judgment when she was young—but that doesn't constitute a sin in my book. In hers, though, I guess it does, since she belongs to one of those conservative sects."

"Carroll, I know you said you're not feeling very compassionate towards her and that makes you a fraud, but on almost every other topic we have ever covered, you're extremely compassionate. Just look at the way you go overboard with those Trollops, and they are not even your clients."

"Well, I don't know, Dr. S. I just don't get it with Blanche."

She looked at her watch and started gathering her papers, putting them in her briefcase with her glasses and date book.

"Oops. Gotta run—catching the late plane out tonight, and I have about a million folks to see in the office today. See you next week—oh, wait, no, I won't see you until after the first of the year."

"I'll be eager to hear what you do about going to Sonoma, Carroll."

Dr. Sutton watched as Carroll's vapor trail slowly disappeared.

"I wish she would slow down and take a deeper look inside herself before she implodes," he muttered softly, as he walked out onto the small patio.

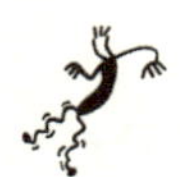

Saturday, Feb, 14, 2004

Park City, Utah

"Mitch, you're a closeted romantic, aren't you?"

Carroll smiled across the table, as they waited for their escargots to be served at Adolph's.

"I can't believe you actually went to the trouble of telling me how you'd tried to get a reservation here three months ago and they were already full on Valentine's, and the only way we could get in would be to stand by, then when we got here tonight, they obviously were expecting us. You are too much."

She reached over and squeezed his hand, looking up just then to see her gray-headed old friend approaching the table.

"Carroll, my dear, so lovely to see you. And Mitch, you're looking well. This relationship must be agreeing with the two of you! Wish I could stay to visit for longer but this is our busiest night of the year."

"Thanks, Adolph. We'll catch you another time."

Devouring the last morsel of the tiny crustacean, then sopping the juices with his bread, Mitch looked across at Carroll and said, "I never would have believed this time last year that I'd be sitting in Adolph's eating snails on Valentine's with someone I adore especially after what happened in Sonoma." He rolled his eyes and Carroll squeezed his hand.

Carroll's eyes brimmed. "I adore you, too, Mitch." *I'm glad he put it that way—love is too big a word for me to say just yet.*

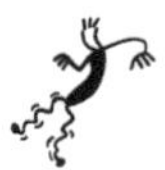

February 17, 2004

——Original message——

To: drcarroll@thesexladyonline.com

From:trixielovesvols@yahoo.com

Subject: Valentines gift

Dear Dr. Carroll:

Well, this is one for the books. I guess it was a good thing I called Troy up last week to remind him Valentine's was coming up right soon—and of course their anniversary, too. Do you know what he went and got Peggy for the big day this year?

Lord, honey, that boy takes the cake. Now you know how I have told you about the way Peggy just loves to garden. Honey, some people have a green thumb, but that cousin of mine, I mean, she has got ten green thumbs. She can make just about anything in the whole wide world grow in that yard of hers. Lord, honey, I wish to heaven you could see her yard in the spring time when all those iris and daffodils and lilacs and all manner of other beautiful blossoms just about knock each other down trying to outdo the ones growing next to them. But anyway, honey, well Troy—now you will remember he has never in his whole entire life ever done one bit of yard work—he's either got allergies or a bad back or some such kind of thing going on. Well, honey, that boy finally got Peggy something she can actually use for once, and guess what it is? After I reminded him about the big day coming up, that Troy got in his red pickup truck and drove himself right down to the Home Depot and told them to load him up with as many bags of manure as they could get in that truck bed, then he came home and piled them right up beside the garage and put a big old red bow on them. When Peggy saw them, she just let out a yell and said, "Oh, shit, Troy, you hit the jackpot this time!" Now if that don't beat all—there she was with 400 pounds of composted manure for her garden, and she called it exactly by its name.

I'll bet she treated Troy real good on Valentine's night, if you get my drift! Ha! Ha!

Your friend,

Trixie

P.S. E.R. gave me a pretty little card that he picked up at Walgreen's for 99 cents—I know 'cause I turned it over and looked at the back.

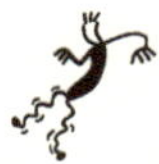

February 29, 2004

--------Original message--------

To: drcarroll@thesexladyonline.com

From: trixielovesvols@yahoo.com

Subject: E.R.

Dear Dr. Carroll:

Oh, honey, just when I didn't think things could get any worse, you won't believe what has happened now. Oh, Lord, I am just too embarrassed to hardly be able to tell you about this one, but I guess if there is one person in the whole wide world who might understand it would be you. So here's what happened.

It was Saturday night, and I just wanted to put my feet up and have a cold margarita. You know, honey, I just almost never drink anymore, except for margaritas. That champagne at Faye and Mark's wedding reception just about put me six feet under and I have sworn off it for the rest of my life. Not that I was ever a heavy drinker or anything. I mean, I could never stand the taste of beer. The only thing I could ever see any good about beer was to put on my hair when I was in my teens and twenties. Lord, honey, if you just let it get about a day or two stale, then you dipped your comb in that brew and ran the comb through your hair before you put your hair up in curlers, then the curl would stay there for days. It was a whole lot cheaper than that Dippity Do stuff and Lord knows, there was enough stale beer sitting around my house when me and Joe were still together, so even if I do say so myself, I kept my hair looking real good back then.

Do you know what that Peggy does with beer? She puts it in small bowls and sets them around in her garden to kill the slugs. Lord, honey, if I tried that, with my luck, some poor old polecat would come along and drink it and then he would just let out a stink, and there I would be, suffocating in this doublewide.

Anyway, I had made myself a margarita and sat down on the divan, and I was feeling about as good as a girl can feel while she is still sober. And then, honey, don't you just know the phone started ringing and when I answered it, it was a collect call from the Nashville jail! I said to myself why would anybody call me collect from the Nashville jail? And then I heard that operator say it was from a Mister Ernest Robert Spalding.

Now, to tell you the truth, honey, it took me about a minute to put two and two together and recognize who she meant. I have never in my life heard anybody call E.R. by anything except those two initials, and I wasn't right sure I knew any Ernest Robert.

But then it sunk in and I said I would accept the call.

And do you know what E.R. said?

Dr. Carroll, he said he had been set up by the police who had been running a sting operation in Centennial Park, and even though his alibi was completely true, they arrested him anyway, and he needed me to come down to the jail and bail him out. I asked him what he was arrested for, and he said he would fill me in later and to come right away and to bring his Bible—the one he always carries with him, but somehow he had forgotten to take it this afternoon.

So I picked that Good Book up off the bedside table and when I did, a little card fell out that I guess he had been using as a bookmark. And Dr. Carroll, I promise you—cross my heart and hope to die—I was not trying to spy on him, but that card fell on the floor just as plain as day, and it said, "Are you bi-curious?" and there was a local phone number underlined.

Well, frankly, Dr. Carroll, I did not know what bi-curious meant so I looked it up in the Webster's, but I guess that dictionary was too old to have the word in it, so then I tried to find out on the Internet, but I ended up getting myself into about a gazillion nasty web sites, so I finally gave up. But by then, I had a pretty good idea what bi-curious meant.

And sure enough, as soon as I got E.R. out of jail and in my car, I looked him straight in the eye and I said, "Are you bi-curious?" Well, honey, bless his heart, you would have thought I had shot a hole clear through him. He just started bawling, and he said he was doing some undercover surveillance for his church group—you know, they are the ones what picket the statue of the naked musicians on Music Row and that Athena statue in the Parthenon and sometimes they picket the adult bookstores. Part of his surveillance was to offer to buy a date with a man in the park, and wouldn't you just know the very man he picked was an undercover Metro cop.

And that cop recognized E.R. from his ambulance work, and he roughed him up a little and said he thought E.R. was the scum of the earth for trying to have sex with a man in the park. And then E.R. lifted up his ball cap and showed me a big ole pump knot on the back of his head.

Oh, Dr. Carroll, this is an awful mess. I just don't know whether to believe E.R. about the surveillance or not. You know, sometimes when he just shows no sexual interest whatsoever in me, I get to wondering if he might be queer. I mean, we are not exactly spring chickens, but we are not yet ready to go to the nursing home either. But then, he has such hate for people who are gay, so I just don't see how he could be one himself.

What do you think I should do?

Your friend,

Trixie

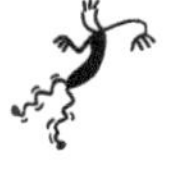

March 1, 2004

Southern California

"Oh, Dr. S., it's so good to see you up and around again. I've been so worried about you." She hugged him gingerly, noticing the vast change in his body size since their last meeting.

"You're wasting away," she said, and immediately regretted her choice of words.

Dr. Sutton's heart problems had worsened over the last three months, and after two hospitalizations and a stay in a nursing home to recuperate, he seemed to have aged ten years since their last supervision session.

"Not to worry, Carroll. I'm not done here yet. Let me get you some tea."

His frailty as he shuffled to the kitchen signaled Carroll to follow him and carry her own steaming cup to the office. For once, the patio door was closed, and she watched him carefully ease himself down in the chair, which seemed to swallow his frame.

"I want to catch up with you, and especially to get an update about Mitch. You may have already told me, but I think my memory is slipping a little with all these medicines I'm on. Did you two go to Sonoma like you mentioned you might when we last met?"

"Oh, yes, we went. It was great and awful at the same time, but things are back on track now, and I had a great Valentine's weekend with him in Park City. For the first time since I've been going there, I didn't rent a condo." She grinned and sipped her tea.

"So you two are finally in the same bed together, huh?"

"Oh, yes. Have been since Sonoma, to tell you the truth. I won't bore you with the details, but let's just say that things almost unraveled on that trip when he tasted just a little too much wine at Chateau St. Jean's, where we spent almost four hours tasting one afternoon. Later, when we tried to make love, he couldn't get an erection, and one would have thought the world was about to end. With a combination of me playing therapist, him sobering up, and some—uhh—assisted loving, we—uhh—got things back up to speed, so to speak, but he did huff around for awhile. It's all better now, thank goodness."

"Well, that's the best news I've had in ages, Carroll." *Smart guy, very smart guy—let her rescue him this time. That trick almost always works!*

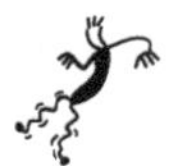

March 3, 2004

To: trixielovesvols@yahoo.com

From: drcarroll@thesexladyonline.com

Subject: Re: E.R.

Trixie,

Yes, I can see how you would think this is an awful mess. What a shock for you! I know E.R. must have been grateful to have you come to his rescue.

This has probably happened for one of three reasons: 1) he is a closeted gay man or a bisexual, meaning he is attracted to both men and women, 2) he is a sex addict and was cruising for a hit, or 3) he was sexually abused sometime in his life and is caught in what we therapists call a repetition compulsion.

I doubt he will think very much of whatever I might say about this, so since you are the one who wants help, maybe you can find a counselor somewhere there to talk to. Ask Peggy—I bet she knows some good therapists from working as a nurse.

Take care of yourself.

Carroll

P.S. I guess there's a fourth reason—maybe he really was doing surveillance work for his church.

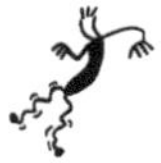

March 4, 2004

Southern California

On the way home from yoga, Carroll stopped by Whole Foods and picked up some tabbouleh and edamame and several bars of organic chocolate. As she and several hundred other shoppers tried to exit the mall, Carroll glanced at the driver in the car next to hers. *Look at her,* she thought, regarding the heavyset woman driving the SUV. *Wonder why a person just lets herself go like that?*

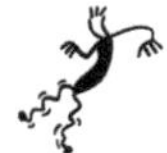

She and Estelle were just hitting the seven-mile mark of their weekly power walk, when Carroll recalled the woman and commented, "Maybe they get it through their genes and maybe they just get worn out from all the burdens of balancing family and career and other activities. For me, if it has four legs don't eat it and if it's white don't bite it."

Estelle smiled, having heard Dr. Carroll's Rules for Life more than once before.

Carroll continued, "But I'm determined not to let myself go to pot, no matter what my family genetic code might be."

"Dr. Carroll Murphy!" Estelle scolded. "Please leave your professional hat at the office and just be a person. Genetic code! For heaven's sake, why can't you just speak plain English?"

Carroll ruefully looked down at her striding feet and agreed. "Sometimes I do struggle to speak plainly. But, believe me, I am getting lots of practice with my new, uh, *clients* in Tennessee. You wouldn't believe some of the messes they get themselves into."

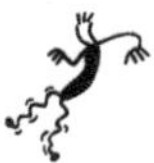

March 5, 2004

To: drcarroll@thesexladyonline.com

From: trixielovesvols@yahoo.com

Subject: Re: Re: E.R.

Dear Dr. Carroll:

I sure hope E.R. was not sexually abused as a child. He would never admit it, if he was. I am sure of that.

Thanks.

Your friend,

Trixie

P.S. They put his picture in the newspaper, along with several other guys they arrested that same day. The story made a big deal about his alibi, like they were making fun of it. I just hate the way those reporters will say whatever they want to in their stories and not even think for a minute about how a body feels. They just do not have any manners.

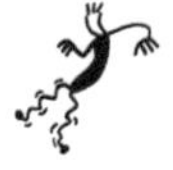

March 6, 2004

Southern California

Carroll had persuaded Estelle to join her in learning to play golf, assuring her walking partner they would never ride in a golf cart when they played if at all possible.

"I can't see why people go to all the trouble to get out and exercise, and then put their clubs on the back of a cart and ride from place to place. It seems to me, walking is where one gets the health benefits of golf," she had lamented to Estelle, who had asked if they could still chat while playing.

Carroll found the talking part difficult. She was so intent on holding her club appropriately and turning her hips through while hitting the ball that she almost never even smiled while she was playing.

As she stood on the tee box, mentally checking off Petra's list—"hands positioned so the V of your right hand is pointed to your right shoulder and your feet are exactly shoulder-width apart"—and seeing the words *coil, recoil* playing on the marquee in her mind, she put her tongue just to right of center on her lips and drew her driver around behind her right shoulder and then pulled it down to strike the ball, which went all of fifty yards to the right before bouncing into the lake.

"Girl, you have got to relax. What's the most important thing you tell your clients to do when they are trying to have better sex?" Estelle asked.

"I tell them to breathe," Carroll answered and grinned, glimpsing momentarily the overlap between good sex and good golf.

"That's right. You need to take your own advice and start breathing. Good grief, you stand there and hold your breath on every shot you take." Estelle chuckled. "My granny used to tell me, 'Estelle, you will never get anywhere except dead if you keep holding your breath,' and you know what, she was absolutely right."

Estelle stepped up to the par-five sixth hole and hit her Big Bertha straight down the fairway 180 yards. "No shit, Granny!" she crowed, and her laugh echoed across two other fairways.

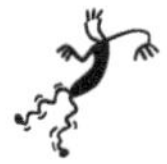

March 18, 2004

Southern California

Send to: trixielovesvols@yahoo.com

You and Peggy want me to come speak to the Trollops A-List Book Club meeting next month during my trip to Nashville? Carroll typed into the IM screen.

"That's right, honey. We would just be tickled pink—or maybe it is tickled red—if you would do this. Every single one of us girls just loves you, and they are so jealous of me and Peggy 'cause we met you in the flesh and blood, and you are practically a member of our family after these past four years of being online buddies. So it would be sort of like a family reunion. And you could meet Faye and Lisa Marie and maybe even Troy. 'Course E.R. won't be there."

O.K., Trixie, I'll do it. It will have to be on the Thursday night I arrive, because my schedule is completely filled for the rest of the time I'm at the conference, but if you can put up with me after I have just flown in from Los Angeles, I will be honored to come to your book club meeting. By the way, do you ever really talk about books?

"Well, I am glad you asked, because we are really and truly going to talk about a book for this meeting. It will be *The Scarlet Letter*."

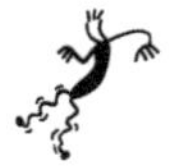

April 19, 2004

Southern California

"Dr. S., they want me to speak to their sorority or book club or whatever they're calling it this week, when I'm in Nashville next month. If it isn't bad enough I have to be in that city—and you know I wouldn't go at all if the sex therapists weren't giving me that award during their convention—but I actually accepted the Trollops' invitation."

Carroll sipped her tea, standing in the doorway from the balcony. The fog still shrouded the shoreline, but she could hear the seals barking furiously.

"Can't you just see it now? Twenty-five women decked out in their white Keds and anklets, probably wearing T-shirts that say 'I am a Trollop' and me trying to talk about a serious work of literature. I think I will throw up!"

Dr. Sutton smiled over his half rims and said, "Well, Carroll, you didn't have to accept their invitation, you know. You could have found all kinds of ways to say no, and they would have gotten along fine without you. So why do you think you said yes?"

"I don't know, Dr. S. I really don't know."

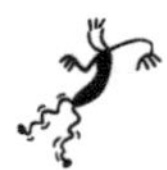

April 30, 2004

--------Original message--------

To: drcarroll@thesexladyonline.com

From: trixielovesvols@yahoo.com

Subject: Mother's Day

Dear Dr. Carroll:

I don't know how I will ever get through these next few weeks. I just cannot imagine having a Mother's Day without having a mother. I mean, of course I have a mother, but she is not—now how can I say this—Lord, honey, she is not here—in person, I mean. Now I know nobody's mother is really here when they have passed, but somehow I just did not think Rainey would ever really be gone. But I guess she has just changed bodies like she always said she wanted to do—you know, honey, from the time she was about seventy years old, she always kept saying to me she was going to hijack the body of some good-looking young thing because the body she was wearing was getting too worn out, and since she had lots more living to do then she thought she would just get herself a new body. She used to say nobody better make her mad, 'cause she was an old woman and that made her mad enough.

Lord, honey, when I went and saw that *Ghostbusters* movie in about 1984, and those spirits kept flying right out of those bodies and then talking to their kin from some other place, I got so shook up that I haven't hardly ever been to a movie since then. So I reckon Rainey's spirit probably did leave her body before we had her cremated, but I don't know where her spirit went. Sometimes I think she has moved inside of me.

Can you believe I am saying this? I mean, I don't think I am possessed or anything, but sometimes I look in the mirror when I am putting on my makeup and oh Lord, honey, there is Rainey staring right back at me.

Anyway, honey, I don't know what you think about all this. Do you ever think about not having a mother when it gets to be this time of the year? I don't mean to pry, but I remember once you said you have been a orphan since you were about seventeen. And if you don't have one single other person in the world you are kin to, that got me to wondering. What do you do on Mother's Day if you don't have a mother?

Your friend,

Trixie

P.S. Me and Peggy will be waiting for you in the baggage area at the bottom of the escalator—they won't let us come to the gate since they think we might be some kind of a terrorist. You will know who we are 'cause we will be waving a sign that says "Trollops (heart) Dr. Carroll!"

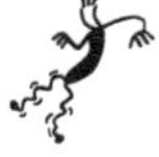

May 2, 2004

To: trixielovesvols@yahoo.com

From: drcarroll@thesexladyonline.com

Subject: Re: Mother's Day

Trixie:

Yes, I know it will be very tough for you to go through this holiday without your mother, but I'm sure you will be just fine. The way I cope with it is I just completely ignore it. It's actually fairly easy for me to do, since I am usually working then anyway.

For you, though, I would suggest you do a couple of things, like making one of Rainey's special recipes, and then maybe you and Peggy could go for a walk, since I bet Troy will be playing golf and she might be lonely too.

Carroll

P.S. I'm looking forward to seeing both of you next week!

Carroll pushed the send key and hoped she would not have to do too much mothering of Trixie when she got there.

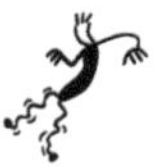

May 3, 2004

———Original message———

To: jrsfreeagain@aol.com

From: drcarroll@thesexladyonline.com

Subject: Chicago

Janie—Crunched for time so I'll catch you up when I see you. I'm planning to leave Nashville right after the awards presentation on Sunday morning, so I'll get into Midway about 4:00. I'll look for you at curbside. It'll be great to see you. Wish I had time for that golf game you mentioned, but by the time I finish taping the show on Monday, I'll have to catch the late plane for L.A.. Maybe next time.

Bye.

Carroll

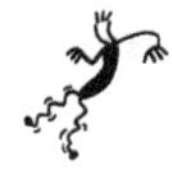

May 5, 2004

Southern California

"You are going to do what?" asked Carroll, breathless with exertion.

"I'm going to take my Harley and ride from Jackson all the way through the Tetons and Yellowstone and go to the Buffalo Bill Museum in Cody, Wyoming, then on to the Black Hills of South Dakota," Mitch said. "I wondered if you'd like to come along on the back of the bike with me."

Carroll grasped the side bars of her treadmill and pushed the pause button. As the rubber mat slowed to a crawl, she stepped to the side rails and from there to the floor. Her brow shimmered with the efforts of her five-mile interval training. She reached for her lime-flavored water and swallowed a large mouthful.

"You have got to be out of your mind. That is a nasty, dangerous hobby and nobody in his right mind would get on one of those monstrosities."

"I beg to differ with you, Dr. Know Everything. Cycles are very safe these days, unless the rider is drinking or not paying attention, and I do not intend to be guilty of either. Surely you have an inner Evel Knievel lurking somewhere, just waiting to be outed," teased Mitch into his cell phone.

"No way. I have a client who lost a leg in a motorcycle accident when he was in college, and I don't wish to risk that kind of gory accident," retorted Carroll, mopping her brow and taking another drag of lime water.

"Well, I won't be having any accidents, and you'll miss out on some glorious scenery. The end of July in Wyoming is stunning, and we'll roar on into Sturgis the first week of August for the biggest rally in the world. Think it over. I think you would look great in leather," he purred.

"I just don't get you," Carroll responded. "First you tell me you want me to learn to play golf because Utah has some of the best public courses in the world and the scenery is terrific. So I think, okay, maybe I can play golf, since it's not violent and the walking is good exercise, then you go and switch sports on me. And the one you choose is so redneck."

"Redneck!" Mitch guffawed. "Redneck! You are going to be up to your ears in rednecks when you go to Tennessee. So don't go calling me a redneck."

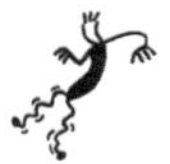

May 6, 2004

Southern California

The morning rush-hour traffic to LAX was worse than usual. Carroll took a last swig of coffee and pulled into a parking place in the overflow lot. In spite of the several hundred people in front of her in the snaking security line, she managed to get to her gate just in time to make her plane to Nashville.

Seated in her aisle seat and breathing deeply, she scanned the parade of other incoming passengers, then opened her cell phone and pushed the number three on her speed dial. After four rings, she heard Mitch's answering machine click on. She bypassed his message and began to speak.

"Hi. Sorry I missed you. This is the only chance I've had to return your call. My session ran late last night, and then I hit major traffic getting to the airport this morning, and you know how I don't like to try to use the phone with that mess going on. Anyway, I'm on the plane now, and they're getting ready to close the cabin door so I'll have to shut down in a minute. I've got an empty seat between me and the window, so maybe I'll finally be able to get the book read without being interrupted. Wish me luck! I'll call you from Nashville later tonight. The Trollops are supposed to meet me at the airport—

well, I hope just two of them will be there—then we'll go straight to their book club. This should be a real experience. I'm beat, and I'll need to get in bed early so I can be ready for tomorrow's session at the conference, so I'll try to get to the hotel by 10:00 or so. Talk to you then. Bye."

Carroll leaned a little into the aisle beside her left leg, letting just a few stray curly hairs cascade across her brow. The seat belt was tangled, and as she twirled it to straighten it out, she glimpsed the boots. Black, scuffed, with heavy chrome chains around the ankles. Trying in vain to conceal the top of the boots were two pant legs of worn denim jeans, the knees of which had given up any chance of offering coverage long ago. As her eyes slowly ascended the figure standing silently in front of her, the watch chain and attached wallet were repositioned by a hambone hand, which then swept upwards to a face wearing a great white beard, guarded in the rear by a gray ponytail. The black T-shirt, sleeves rolled almost to the armpits, somewhat covered the ample belly that oozed out under the black leather vest. STURGIS, screamed the embroidered patch on one side of the vest front; the distinctive Harley-Davidson crest on the back was visible as he reached to stow a backpack above the seats across from Carroll.

"I believe that's my seat, ma'am," he said, pointing to the empty one next to Carroll.

No way. This cannot be happening again to me, Carroll thought, swaying slightly as she stood and moved into the aisle to make room for his descent.

The petite, drably dressed woman sitting next to the window smiled politely, then turned her head toward the glass panel, watching the line of luggage being delivered into the underbelly of the plane.

He spilled his girth across both sides of his seat, poking about with his massive hands to locate the two ends of the seat belt.

"Looks like some little feller was sitting here before," he declared, before letting the belt out its full length and buckling it tight.

Carroll wondered whether that belt could really hold so much personhood if a sudden stop were made.

Probably he would just bounce off the front seat and splatter, but no damage would be done, she guessed.

"I've been to a rally, honey. Ever been to one of those?" He tossed the question to either woman, hoping he might get lucky.

"That's not for me, I'm afraid," the luggage watcher answered.

"Well, now, don't knock it if you haven't tried it, that's what I say. I'm Ronnie, honey. What's your name?"

The hambone extended, and the woman's tiny hand seemed almost lost as she met his handshake and mumbled, "Shirley."

"What do you do for a living, if I might be so bold?"

"I'm a church youth director," she barely whispered.

"Well, bless your heart. Ain't that something about all them youth preachers getting themselves tangled up in porn sites on the Web?" He turned to Carroll. "And what about you, honey?"

"I'm a sex therapist," she answered, immediately regretting this self-revelation.

"No shit!" crowed Ronnie. "My buddies ain't gonna believe I sat between the church lady and a for-sure lady sex therapist all the way from L.A. to Nashville. Ain't that the cat's meow!" He slapped his knee for emphasis, letting little tornadoes of road dust loose with each blow.

"Can I ask you something?" he said, leaning into what little space Carroll could call her own. "Is it normal to chase women?"

Knowing from experience he wasn't so much wanting an answer as to have an opportunity to tell more of his story, Carroll did not respond.

"I'm fifty-five years old and I got me a wife about the same age. I used to be a workaholic—I owned a little chain of pawn shops, don't you know—but then I hit fifty, and I just decided to quit work and chase women. Now my wife, she don't seem to care. She says as long as I don't bring nothing home that's catching, it don't bother her a bit what I do. So I decided to ride Harleys and see the USA."

Shirley pulled out her Bible and started reading. Carroll wished she had a Bible to read for herself right now. The only things in her briefcase were professional journals and a copy of *The Scarlet Letter*.

"I used to weigh 360 pounds, but then I had my stomach stapled. It didn't help my weight too much, but it did help my high blood pressure and my diabetes."

Ronnie turned his massive head to check out the impression he was making on Carroll, whose eyes were now partially closed.

"Do you know what the cure for tendinitis is? Mattress mambo! I don't hardly ever get sore any more when I do that kind of dancing," he laughed. "I don't do no drugs, mind you. No sirree, none of that freaky stuff for me. I just go to those rallies, and every afternoon about four o'clock I just sit myself down and wait for the tit parade to come by."

Carroll closed her eyes tightly, hoping for sleep, or at least a good imitation of slumber.

"Hey, guess what? Hey, you're not listening. Guess what? My testosterone level is more than 850. My doctor said he had never seen those kind of results in any of his patients. What do you think about that?"

Nodding, Carroll acknowledged his world-class number and put her head back again.

"You know what, though? Old age sucks. Everything that's supposed to be limber gets hard, and everything that's supposed to be hard gets limber."

Without opening her eyes, Dr. Carroll mentally catalogued the new phrase into the archives.

"Well, I guess it's better than being in prison, though. That's where my daughter is—in the penitentiary. She killed a man in my home. She did it all right. She was on drugs. I can't excuse her behavior, though, even if she is my own kin."

Carroll never opened her eyes again for the three and one half hours into Nashville airspace. For all she knew, Ronnie had talked the whole way. She awakened to hear him telling her he tried to be good to his sister, who was on oxygen.

"I try not to be gone from home too long at a time because I take her to Walmart every week of her life. But do you know what?"

"No, what?" Carroll responded on cue, keeping her eyes closed.

"I don't think we can ever take her on no airplane trip nowadays since that ValuJet crashed into the Everglades. See, they won't let you bring your own oxygen on board now, and she says she for sure will not travel with somebody else's air because she just don't trust it. If that don't beat all."

Nodding groggily as the flight attendant signaled the arrival in Nashville, Carroll began to search around her seat for anything she might have brought aboard.

Ronnie's hand invited a shake from her and Carroll endured one more piece of his life wisdom.

"You sure are a good-looking gal. I bet you ain't never used no cigarettes or gotten any suntans. Lord, those two things can ruin a girl's looks when she gets older."

Carroll nodded, and then she squeezed into the crowded aisle and crept to the open door with the rest of her fellow travelers. Starting up the corridor to the passenger exit, she took one more swallow of her lime water and wondered if she could wing it with the Trollops without having read *The Scarlet Letter* since her college English class forty years ago.

She ducked into the restroom and used the facilities, checking her hair and lipstick in the mirror before exiting with the female throngs. Riding down the escalator to the baggage section, she wobbled a little as she was welcomed to Music City by several lighted homespun signs over her head offering the joys of the Grand Ole Opry and Cracker Barrel restaurants. The scent of English Rose reached her first, and then she heard Trixie and Peggy calling her name. *I am definitely descending into Trollop hell.*

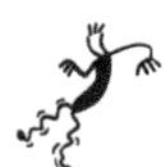

As they rounded the corner into Peggy's subdivision, Trixie shrieked and pointed to the hand-painted bed sheet draped over the brick-framed sign indicating the entrance to Camelot Downs. WELCOME DR. CARROLL. FRESH FROM OPRAH TO MT. JULIET!

"Well, I never," purred Trixie. "I knew it was a right friendly neighborhood, but I sure didn't expect that kind of welcome. What do you think about that, Dr. Carroll?"

Carroll kept her true thoughts bundled tightly inside, as she politely smiled and nodded. "Well, it certainly does seem like southern hospitality," she replied.

Both cousins smiled and squeezed each other's hands across the console.

Approaching 401 Guinevere Drive, they saw cars lining both sides of the street. In the doorway of Peggy's modest ranch home stood three women holding a bouquet of balloons and scanning the horizon. As they glimpsed the steel-blue SUV turning into the driveway, they burst forth and behind them swarmed at least fifteen others, all wearing white tennis shoes and white anklets, all tittering and grinning.

The Publisher's Clearing House van has arrived to award the $100,000 grand prize check, Carroll thought. For a moment she hesitated getting out of the door which was already being opened by one of the women. Her stomach turned and she felt a momentary panic rise in her throat. *Please let me get through this in one piece*, she prayed to the Universe.

Then Dr. Carroll Murphy painted on her smile, shook her auburn curls, and stepped one then another well-shod foot out of the backseat of Peggy's Blazer and was transformed into the media maven for whom all this audience was waiting. Shaking hands all around, she nodded and quipped to each woman, hitting her stride as Peggy presented to her a lovely thirty-something woman she introduced as "my little Lisa Marie."

"Well, since she's just about to turn thirty-six, she's not so little any more, but I guess in my mind she'll always be my little girl," Peggy gushed.

"I'm very pleased to meet you, Lisa Marie," said Carroll, looking directly into Lisa Marie's cobalt-blue eyes, which were framed by the darkest, longest lashes Carroll had ever seen. "I've certainly heard a lot about you over the years from your mother." Carroll could not be sure, but just for an instance she felt some flutter of kinship with Lisa Marie.

"And I've heard lots about you, too, Dr. Carroll," laughed Lisa Marie. "Since Mother met you, I don't think any decisions have been made in our house unless she has run the problem by you."

Both women smiled at the memory of all the Internet traffic that had passed between Carroll and Peggy in the last few years.

They walked on into the house, entering Peggy's living room, which adjoined the dining area at the rear of the house. Carroll thought she glimpsed a male figure outside standing next to a huge kettle style grill and looking in through the sliding glass doors to the patio, but when she looked back he was not there. Trixie nudged her elbow and whispered in her ear, "There's Faye over by the mantel. She's the one in the glider rocker. She's feeding Moses."

Trixie's pearlized acrylic nail pointed across the room to the white chair in which was seated an oval-faced young woman, with long brown hair pulled away from her face and clipped up at the crown. As Carroll's eyes swept Peggy's tidy living room, they landed on the young mom, whose baby was happily guzzling a bottle. Carroll strained to recognize any likeness between Trixie and her daughter.

Trixie noted Carroll's puzzled look and offered, "She takes more after her daddy's side of the family, rest his soul, than mine, honey."

"Did you say Moses, Trixie? I thought you said the baby had been named after your father, Floyd."

"Well, honey, that's what I thought, too, but she and Mark decided Floyd was too plain a name, and they started calling him by his middle name about two weeks ago. It's kind of hard for me to get used to it, but I just think of him like that little Israelite baby whose mama had to put him in a basket of rushes or he would be killed, and then he was found by the princess, and I think it fits pretty well, since this little Moses was also adopted."

Carroll's knees weakened for a moment, and feeling herself get a little light-headed, she asked her hostess for a glass of water.

"Sure, sweetie."

Peggy quickly returned from the kitchen, saying, "Here you have the finest Tennessee tap water we can offer. Bound to restore your soul."

Carroll drank slowly, draining the glass. *What is going on with me?* Surely she was just reacting to all the commotion surrounding her arrival in Tennessee and the hoopla at Peggy's house. But there was some nagging feeling in her gut that seemed like the sensation she had heard other women describe when they discover they are pregnant. Sort of a cross between fatigue and nausea, mixed with some anticipation and wonder. *Couldn't be that*, Carroll smiled wanly. *Not possible after five years of menopause.*

The book club ladies had almost emptied the table of munchies by the time Peggy and Trixie called them to order in the living room. Faye had removed the now-contented Moses from his bottle and handed him to her mother. Carroll moved to her designated seat of honor on Peggy's kitchen stool next to Faye, and they chatted briefly, with Carroll promising Faye they would get better acquainted after the book discussion. Faye nodded in agreement and looked lovingly at the sleeping Moses in Trixie's arms.

Peggy stood to welcome the ladies to their monthly meeting and asked Martha to deliver the opening prayer. Peggy noted they had some new business to conduct before Trixie introduced their special guest.

Carroll remembered Trixie having told her that for the first couple of years, as the Trollops were still figuring out what they were about, their meetings were basically just to gather and talk. One day a new member brought in a local story about the way the right-to-lifers, as she called them, were picketing the Planned Parenthood where abortions were carried out.

The Trollops had a silent rule never to try to influence anyone's beliefs about what to do in the event of an unintended pregnancy. "Lord, honey, if we let ourselves get into that bag of worms, we would have more scratching than in a hen house," Trixie had told Joan by e-mail.

"But I think the Trollops have a lot in common with those girls who go to Planned Parenthood, so maybe you all could do a little something for them," Joan had offered from her perspective in Michigan.

At the next meeting, a box was set up for anybody who wanted to donate any things that would help a new mother with a baby get on her feet, and before long, the Trollop Triplets sorority had become a service group along with being a book club.

Peggy acknowledged Maribeth, their service representative, who told the ladies, "With this being the week before Mother's Day and all the hoopla that goes along with that holiday, we thought it would be a good idea to support Birth Mother's Day, a new holiday, which takes place the day before Mother's Day. There will be a picnic in Centennial Park on Saturday and I hope lots of you will show up. We each need to bring a covered dish that will feed eight people. Sweet tea and milk will be provided, but we need paper plates and drink cups."

She passed a sign-up list, and soon it was covered with names and pledged offerings of food and service implements.

I cannot believe this, Carroll thought. There seemed to be such a genuine show of concern and affection, not only for each girl and woman in the room, but also for the unnamed girls and women cited as subjects for their caring. In her experience in Los Angeles and in the other domains where she was a public figure, she would often hear celebrities expounding on the charity of their choice, but almost always she found their care to be detached and probably scripted for the public's consumption, having little to do with the reality of their lives.

While the sign-up list was circulating, Trixie held the sleeping Moses, talking both to him and to Carroll without lifting her gaze from her grandson.

"Moses, honey, now this may not be politically correct to say—and you know I am as much in favor of helping out those birth mothers as the next person—but I sure do hope you don't decide one day to go looking for your birth mother."

She handed him back to Faye so she could start her introduction, turning to Carroll with one more thought.

"Why is it today that these young 'uns cannot just be okay with the parents what raised them up? There they are with every single little thing in the whole wide world they could want, and they have to get on the Internet and start searching all over the place for the daddy and mama what made them. If that don't beat all!"

Carroll swayed but steadied herself with her hand on the edge of the seat and swigged some more water.

Trixie stood to address the club members, tapping her spoon against the side of her glass of Diet Coke to get their attention.

"Ladies, I know you are all excited to be here tonight to help Peggy and me welcome Dr. Carroll Murphy of Los Angeles and the Oprah show to the monthly meeting of the Music City Trollop's A-List Book Club."

All twenty women in the room clapped appreciatively, and Moses stirred a little at the noise.

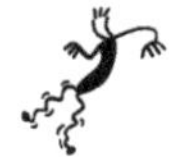

Trixie had typed out her introduction over the last week and had sent it back and forth to Peggy for review. She had never had any experience speaking before an audience and did not want to flub her lines on this one occasion. She told Peggy she knew she would never get to go to the Oscars or the Emmys, which she watched faithfully on TV, nor would she ever get to be Miss America—or in the case of someone her age, Mrs. America—but she thought speaking before the Music City Trollops A-List Book Club might be her one claim to fame.

Trixie's performance was Oscar-worthy. She asked Calvin to be her clothing and hair consultant, and he readily agreed.

"Now I don't want to be too gussied up and make all the other girls feel underdressed, but after all we do have a special guest from California, and I don't want to be embarrassed by looking too plain Jane," she confided to her eldest son.

"Trixie, there's not a chance in the world you would ever look plain Jane," Calvin answered. "There's not been a morning of your life since I have been around, and it's been almost forty-eight years, that the very first thing you have done as soon as your eyes begin to open is to start putting on your makeup. Do you remember when Rainey was about on her deathbed in the hospital and you had come to sit with her, and you forgot to grab your makeup bag and I had to drive twenty-five miles each way from Nashville to Fairview to get it?"

"Yes, honey, I remember. But a girl has to do what a girl has to do. And, honey, it has been so long since I've seen the roots of this hair or my natural face in the sunlight that I would be about scared to death to see them."

Calvin agreed. He accepted long ago that the first and only action, should he be called to identify her body, would be to arrange her hair and to reapply her makeup, so helping her to get ready for her evening in the spotlight, as she started calling her book club appearance, was a no-brainer for Calvin.

He arranged to give her a courtesy hair highlight at the spa, followed by a facial, and then he consulted with her on applying her makeup. Through trial and error, Trixie had become a makeup artist in her own right, so Calvin basically just suggested a little more toner or a little less eye shadow and left his mother to her own artistry. Indeed, his own career in cosmetology had begun in his mother's bedroom when he was about five years old. He got into her makeup bag and began to experiment with applying her cosmetics to his younger brothers.

At first, they were eager for his attention, but when he painted Walter's fingernails with hot pink polish and Walter came home from kindergarten crying because some other boys had called him a fag, Trixie told Calvin he should just stick with applying makeup to himself. She carefully showed him how to remove it with Pond's cold cream and tissues, which she said was always the best thing you could do for your face. And as an adult, Calvin became a favorite makeup artist to many of the country music stars in Nashville, every one of whom got the customary Pond's treatment before and after their gigs.

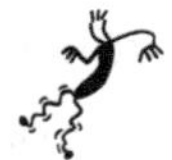

As Trixie stood before the Trollops' A-List Book Club, getting ready to read her lines to introduce Dr. Carroll Murphy, she could have easily passed for a star on the Opry. She debated about wearing her white canvas Keds with the white anklets, but she knew all the other women in the club would be wearing theirs so she followed suit. It had become customary, even for the women who were not originally from East Tennessee, to adopt this particular kind of footwear after becoming Trollops. In fact, it was the only almost-required item of dress in their wardrobe.

"Now, ladies, tonight Dr. Carroll Murphy is going to lead our discussion of *The Scarlet Letter*, by Nathaniel Hawthorne." Trixie stumbled over the last two words, but congratulated herself silently that she had not mixed up the name again as she had while rehearsing with Peggy the previous night.

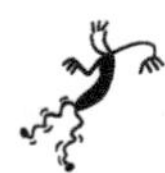

"I don't know why that name is so hard for me to say, honey," she had complained to Peggy.

"That's okay, sweetie," Peggy consoled. "That name about cracked us up in high school English class. Miss Braddock had a hard enough time leading the discussion about the book every year, since I am sure she was still a virgin at her death, but then when our school principal's name was Mr. Hawthorne, too, she nearly choked when she said it."

"Oh, Lord, honey, I do remember Mr. H. It was him what told Rainey and me I couldn't come back to school anymore after I started showing with Calvin. And there I was, just a few weeks shy of finishing the first semester of 12th grade. He looked down his nose at me like he smelled a dead possum. I guess he kind of forgot that his own sweet Earline had given birth to a baby whose daddy was a mystery just a couple of years before."

"And then, Trix, do you remember what we girls did? I mean, I was only in the ninth grade then, but some of your twelfth-grade girlfriends and I snuck over to his house and put some of those pink flamingos, which had been in his neighbor's flower garden, on his lawn. He never did find out who did it!"

"Lord, yes, honey, I remember. 'Course I couldn't go with you all since I was about to give birth and all, but I was sure tickled you got to go along with some of the other twelfth graders to set him straight."

"We were ahead of our time, Trix. Did you know these days you can call up and order a whole flock of those flamingos to be set up in somebody's yard, and the only way to get them removed is for the person to make a donation to the designated charity."

"Lord, honey, what will they think of next?"

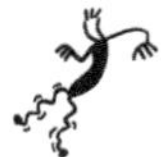

"So, ladies. I am sure all of you have read our monthly book—even though I will just go ahead and confess right now that I have not read it, but I know you all will still love me in the morning anyway—and you will have lots to discuss with Dr. Carroll, who is our red-letter guest, but I don't mean by that a scarlet A." Trixie giggled and sat down, and the rest of the book club ladies glanced around in embarrassment. They knew Trixie had ad-libbed after all.

Carroll again felt that now familiar knot tighten in her stomach. She was barely aware that Lisa Marie had asked her a question.

"I'm sorry, Lisa Marie. I was a little distracted. Jet lag, I guess," she ruefully explained.

Nervous laughter from the audience subsided, and Lisa Marie asked again.

"What do you think it is about an unmarried woman getting pregnant that brings up so much feeling both for and against it in society, Dr. Carroll?"

Reaching for her almost-empty glass of Tennessee tap water, Carroll swallowed a sip and cleared her throat, then she smiled confidently to her audience.

"Well, I guess folks believe every baby conceived has a stake in keeping the society alive by passing down genetic and cultural traditions. So people seem to line up on one side or the other according to whether they think the conceived child has a right to life, or whether the mother has the right to choose to end the pregnancy."

It was a question she had been asked hundreds of times, on call-in radio and TV shows, in front of live audiences, and in her newspaper column and e-mail forum. Years ago, she had perfected the answer in a mock TV studio where she had undergone several rounds of media training.

"Well, what you said may be true," replied Lisa Marie, "but I just can't help thinking if my Aunt Trixie had had a choice when she was sixteen, she might not have had Calvin, and if Mama and Daddy had not got married back in 1968 after I was on the way and Mama had had to raise me as a single mom, or if Faye had not been able to adopt little Moses after his birth mother had chosen to give him up . . . or if I had not got drunk and pregnant by my then-boyfriend and had an abortion when I was a freshman in college, how would things have been different for each one of us. All of this is such a personal situation, and none of us deserves to be labeled with a scarlet A."

Before she could blink hard enough to stop the tears, big drops began to fall from Carroll's eyes. Her audience, silenced by what they were witnessing, saw her body begin to heave, as years of bottled-up emotions broke through the small cracks in her dammed-up spirit. She tried to control herself in all the ways she had used for the past forty years, but none would click in place. As she sat on Peggy's kitchen stool in this ordinary ranch house in Tennessee, three days before Mother's Day, surrounded by twenty women who all had stories of their own, her dam broke.

"What is it, honey?" asked Trixie mouthing to Peggy to fetch the Kleenex from the kitchen. She moved herself instinctively closer to Carroll. "Did one of us say something that hurt your feelings?" She shot a look to Lisa Marie, who had been speaking just before this dam broke. "Oh, honey, we wouldn't want to upset you for all the tea in China."

"Aunt Trixie, I don't think it was me who upset her," Lisa Marie said quietly.

Trixie's arms encircled Carroll's heaving shoulders as she alternated patting and fanning her, while Peggy supplied tissues and more water. The audience sat in stony silence, stealing embarrassed glances at their famous speaker, whose shoes now were dangling at the end of her well manicured toes. Faye reached over and slipped the Bally pumps off Carroll's feet and neatly placed them beside her chair. Moses stirred and whimpered, and Faye stood to take him to his crib in Peggy's guest room.

Lisa Marie stood in front of Carroll, gently but firmly breaching the protective circle that Trixie had fostered. She reached for Carroll's quivering chin with both of her hands and lifted the reluctant face to a level with her own. "Carroll, can you tell us what's happening?" she asked, trying to look directly into Carroll's eyes.

Stuttering uncharacteristically, Carroll's moisture-clogged voice choked out between sobs, "I-I-I'm a Trollop, t-too."

Hushed by this revelation, the group of Trollop sisters began to gather their chairs closer around Carroll. Her sudden break in character type gave them permission to encircle her rather than to sit in front of her, and they waited expectantly for their next cue.

"I-I-I had a baby. Almost forty years ago. A little g-girl. A girl. She was beautiful." More sobs racked Carroll's body, and both Trixie and Peggy hugged her. Lisa Marie held Carroll's hands tightly, as her nails dug into Lisa Marie's palms. Surprisingly, Carroll's stiff body softened enough for all of them to move a little closer.

"I got one look at her, and then I never saw her again. The nuns who ran the home for unwed mothers where I was staying had already made me sign the papers giving her up for adoption." Carroll's pain enveloped her, and she sobbed so loudly that Troy peeked in from the backyard to see if everything was under control. Peggy waved him off and he shrugged his shoulders, puzzled to see the honored guest in such a state of discomposure.

"It's okay, honey. You *are* really one of us." Trixie pointed to her heart, and then motioned to two of her sisters to go to the kitchen.

With little question about what Trixie was signaling, they reappeared in less than five minutes with a trimmed remnant of a Krispy Kreme doughnut box. They had scavenged in Peggy's everything-drawer and located scissors and some magic markers, and in their hands now was a fairly good enlarged replica of the Trollops emblem: a white background with the three Greek letters, Theta Theta Theta, in red, and the year 1998 under the Greek symbols. On the back, the sisters had attached some strapping tape folded over to be double sticky.

Solemnly, Maribeth and Martha, shadowed by the rest of the group, approached Carroll and presented her with their sisterhood emblem. She slowly looked up into their loving, warm eyes and tentatively accepted their gift. Just as she began to attach it to her Kelly green cashmere cardigan, she heard the first strands of Rocky Top emanating from the stereo in the corner. Momentarily horrified, she felt each of her hands being gently taken by Trixie and Peggy as they urged her to join the group, who had begun to buck dance to the Vol Nation anthem.

Hardly believing her own reality, Carroll felt her feet begin to shuffle-step-back-step, then she began to add a little skipping motion, like she had done in her childhood when she and her girlfriends had twirled a jump rope. She resisted for a moment, as her Trollop sisters urged her into the center of the circle and began to clap the sides of their thighs to the cadence of Rocky Top.

"Come on, honey. You can do it. It's therapy for your broken heart," Trixie urged.

When the song ended, most of the Trollop sisters began to make their way to the kitchen to round up their empty plates. Maribeth edged up to Trixie and asked, "Do you think she is going to be okay?"

"Why, sure, honey. She just needs to get herself fluffed up a little and then Peggy and me will drive her right over to that big old Opryland Hotel." She squeezed Maribeth's hand for emphasis, and Maribeth leaned down and patted Carroll's hand. "We love you, Sugar."

Carroll managed to smile back and return the pat.

Martha leaned over and patted Carroll's shoulder. "We'll be praying for you, Honey," she said.

Carroll smiled briefly and patted her back.

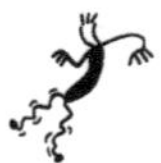

"Well now, that was what I call a meeting we'll all remember," Peggy noted, helping Faye get Moses' diaper bag and bottles into the car while Faye strapped him into the baby seat.

"Who would have thought?" Faye said to Lisa Marie, who smiled.

The three women huddled by the curb, exchanging hugs, then Faye and Lisa Marie drove off and Peggy walked back into her house.

"Is it safe for me to come in yet?" Troy asked, peeking through the partially opened sliding-glass doors. "It looked like you all were having some kind of female commotion in here. What happened?"

"Shhh. She's still here—in there in our bathroom with Trixie," Peggy answered.

"What in hell are they doing in there? Is she teaching Trix some new sex move from California?" Troy laughed.

"No, I can't tell you about it right now, but something really big just happened. Trixie is getting her presentable so we can take her on to her hotel."

Troy couldn't imagine what she meant, but he grabbed a few leftover chips and some salsa, settled himself on his recliner, and pushed the Tivo remote.

"Well, I'm glad to know you are not keeping her here for the night," he said. "But I sure would like to at least shake that woman's hand."

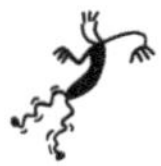

"Lord, honey, you could have knocked me over with a feather when you said you were one of us. I would never in the world have believed it if I hadn't heard it directly from your mouth."

Carroll was sitting on a small stool in front of the plate-glass mirror in Peggy and Troy's master bath, with her head reclined back into Trixie's abdomen.

"Now, honey, you have got to just hold these cucumber slices in place for five minutes and they will take the swelling right out of those eyes of yours. Just lean your head back so they won't fall off and I will massage your temples at the same time, then we'll dab a little powder on your nose and get your wild hair under control, and by the time we get you to that big old hotel, won't anybody know what you have been through."

Trixie was as good as they get on repair jobs after all her years of both personal and professional beauty-maintenance work. "Lord, honey, I am just about a expert in making a silk purse out of a sow's ear," she told Carroll, who was too drained to respond, much less protest.

Peggy came in holding a cup of hot Lipton tea and handed it to Carroll, who lifted the vegetables from her eyes and sat up, accepting it gratefully.

I would never touch this stuff back home, she thought, then surprised herself by noting how good its warmth and taste actually was.

"Now, honey, do you want to tell us more about that little girl of yours, or are you going to keep us in suspense for the rest of our days?" asked Trixie.

Carroll swallowed slowly, then began. "I don't know exactly what to say. I was not quite even eighteen when she was born—August 22, 1964—nine months to the day after Kennedy was shot. I got one look at her and then I turned her over to those nuns. The last I saw of her one of them was holding a crucifix over her head and saying something in Latin."

"Well, excuse me for noticing, honey, but I don't think you got yourself pregnant all by yourself, so who was the daddy?"

Carroll choked on her tea and a little fluid drizzled down her chin and over her new sorority pin onto her sweater. Peggy went to the laundry room to get some spot remover.

"You'd better take that top off and let me take care of it before it permanently sets. It's too good a sweater to get ruined right here."

Reluctantly, Carroll raised her arms and removed the twin set and Peggy handed her a Fan Fair T-shirt out of her closet. They all giggled when they saw Carroll transformed into a typical tourist, and then they put her makeshift sorority pin in place over her heart.

"I have never told this to a soul," she started.

Trixie and Peggy leaned against the Formica cabinet tops and gave her their full attention.

"The night of Kennedy's assassination, I was so upset. I had really believed Camelot was on the horizon and then—*poof*—it was gone. And I felt so bad for Caroline and John, because I knew exactly what it would be like to grow up without a daddy there. So when my Western Civ professor—Robert Barkley, I will never forget his name—when he suggested to me we go to his apartment and have something to help us feel better, I was glad to go. I mean, nothing on campus was normal that night, and I knew it would be no use to call my mother for commiseration—she would either be at work or she would tell me to be strong and I did not feel like being strong just then."

Carroll sipped her tea and Peggy and Trixie looked at each other with slightly raised eyebrows.

"Well, little did I know he would offer me a Scotch and water—which I had never tasted—I mean, I had only just turned seventeen years old . . . I was a year younger than most freshmen because I had skipped first grade, and except for my mother's Jack Daniel's, I had never been around alcohol. But looking back, I think I had a crush on Dr. Barkley—practically all the freshman girls did, too, I think. He told me to call him Robert, and it really felt grown-up to say that word to his face. He had the most impeccable manners; it was always 'please this' and 'thank you that' and about every sentence he said either started or ended with 'ma'am.' To this day I almost get sick at my stomach when somebody says 'ma'am' to me."

She paused and the cousins nodded, then she went on with her story.

"I couldn't stand the taste of that stuff—the Scotch—but I was already a pretty good actress, so I pretended like it was the best-tasting liquid I had ever put into my mouth, and then after the second drink, I started to feel a real buzz and I don't remember much afterwards, except that just before curfew, I remember him telling me we needed to get our clothes back on so I could get to the dorm before it closed."

"Dammit! Men are all the same," Peggy said, thumping her fist on the countertop before looking at Trixie, who knew the source of the comment. One of Peggy's professors from graduate school had tried a similar version of exploitation on her when she was almost fifty years old. She had reported him, and he had been disciplined by the Faculty Senate, to her great satisfaction.

"Then, for the rest of the weekend, I mooned around in my dorm room writing Robert and Mrs. Robert Barkley and Professor and Mrs. Robert Barkley all over pieces of paper. My roommate, Melinda, was out on dates, of course—nobody ever asked me out because I wasn't pretty or rich or southern—so I could just about have done anything and it wouldn't have mattered to the world."

"Carroll, where did this all take place?" Peggy asked.

"Right here in good old Music City USA. I went to Warfield for my freshman year. I wasn't on any birth control—hell, it was my first time—and I knew for sure by Christmas I was pregnant. After I came back to Nashville from Thanksgiving break, he started treating me just like I was any other student. I tried to tell him I thought I was pregnant once when I saw him going into the student center, but then I saw him cuddle up in there with Trish-the-dish from the same Western Civ class, and I knew he would deny it. And back then there was no such thing as DNA proof. So I finished the semester, and then I withdrew from Warfield and left Nashville and I made up my mind never to come back, and until tonight I *had* never come back."

Peggy and Trixie blinked and cut a glance at each other.

"Well, honey, I can see why you might think we don't have any manners here in Middle Tennessee."

Carroll glanced up at Trixie and smiled, reaching for Trixie's hand.

"No, Trixie, I don't think that. I just think Robert Barkley was a world-class jerk."

"Well, he was," agreed Peggy.

"So didn't your mama figure out something was going on with you when you were home for Christmas, Carroll?" asked Peggy

"No, she worked all the time, and I managed to act just like everything was fine. That's the way we always had treated each other. She had no idea what I was going through."

"Well, what happened that you stopped talking to or seeing her? Was it because she did find out later? Lord, that Rainey, she sniffed me out every single time, just about as soon as I even got pregnant."

"No, she never knew. Still doesn't, as far as I know. She had worked a double on Christmas night, and when she came in later than usual in the morning, I was up and sitting at the table trying to eat something. I was already having a little morning sickness, so about all I could stand was toast and tea, but she didn't notice. She headed straight for her Jack Daniel's and sat down at the table and started telling me about her night.

'I swear, Carroll,' she said between gulps. 'This is one Christmas I don't ever want to see again. We had this fifteen-year-old girl brought in by her mother, and she was in labor. She said she didn't even know she was pregnant, and here she was almost six months along—and then she had this awful precipitous delivery right there in the emergency room, and of course the baby died. It was a blessing, I think. That girl's name may have been 'Eileen' but if my daughter had done that, in my book her name would always be 'Slut.' After what she did to her family's good name. I think she deserved what she got."

When she said those words to me, I felt like my heart had just been wrapped in steel, and I knew from that moment on, I would never again have a mother. I hung out at my friend Janie's most of the rest of the break, then went back to Warfield on the train and finished out the semester. I got an A in Western Civ." Carroll looked up and smiled at Peggy and Trixie and they grinned back.

"I packed up all my school things and went back to Evanston and got what I needed from the house at a time when I knew she would be working. I left her a note telling her I was going to find myself in Oregon and for her to not contact me. She would always pry my address out of Janie over the next ten years, but I guess she finally gave up after that because I never answered any of her letters, and that was the last contact I have ever had with her. I do know she is still living, though, because Janie told me so recently."

"Whew! Do you mean to tell me that at seventeen-years-old you moved yourself to Oregon and had your baby and put her up for adoption and finished college, and you did it all by yourself?" asked Peggy, wide-eyed.

"That's about it. I just put one foot in front of the other one and kept plugging along. I waited tables and even tended bar for a while to make ends meet. Oregon accepted me as a special student for the spring term and then after I had the baby I started in as a full-time student for the fall term. Luckily, I had a good mind and could work hard, and I could go pretty far in life on those assets. And now here I am forty years later."

"So have you ever heard from that little girl?" asked Trixie.

Carroll inhaled deeply and shifted on the chair. She fastened her gaze on her painted toenails and spoke quietly. "No. I've thought a few times about signing up for one of those databases that let each person check to see if the other one wants to be contacted, but then I would just put it out of my mind. I have no idea what happened to her, and at this point in my life, with her being almost forty and me approaching sixty, I don't think there's probably much chance either of us would try to do anything. But it doesn't mean I have not thought about her every single day since she was born."

Carroll quietly imploded in tears and Trixie hugged her close, mopping and patting and stroking. After a few minutes of sobbing, Carroll pulled away from Trixie and leaned her head forward between her knees, letting her unruly curls fall forward, breathing in the lingering scent of English Rose, which had penetrated her hair.

"Well, a body just never knows about such things, I guess, honey. What do you reckon ever happened to that old Warfield professor?" asked Trixie.

Carroll sat upright again, looking at herself for the first time in the mirror. She tucked an errant curl back in place and shook her head. "I have no idea. I hope never to see him or to cross paths with him again in this life."

Trixie moved back behind Carroll and began to stroke her hair gently with a brush, wadding a hair band around the red curls to make a ponytail. Carroll shut her eyes and let herself be coiffed, enjoying the peacefulness of the quiet for a moment.

After a few minutes, Trixie piped up, holding the brush in midair.

"Girls, have I got an idea! Let's see if that old buzzard still lives here in Nashville—you can just about track down anybody on the Internet. If he does, let's don't get mad—let's flock him!"

"Flock him? What's that?" asked Carroll, her eyes popping open to the view of Trixie and her hairbrush weapon. The color drained from her face, and she could only imagine what might be involved in this kind of Appalachian revenge crime.

"Oh, honey, a swarm of pink plastic flamingos will land in his yard!"

"Oh . . ."

"And we'll make him pay ransom to the Birth Mothers group!" added Peggy, doubling over at the idea.

Carroll stood up slowly, looking from Peggy to Trixie and back again. Her cheeks began to glow and her eyes narrowed. Her voice became sinister, while her hands carefully framed the next scene.

"Then we'll put up a big sign in his yard, painted in red letters, saying, 'Courtesy of Alpha Chapter of the Trollops Triplets Sorority, assisted by the Bawdy Broads and the Flamingo Girls—colonized at the Redneck College of Sex Nashville campus: May 2004!'".

All three sisters hugged each other, laughing until it was hard to tell whether the tears came from pain or from joy. For once, Carroll did not try to analyze it.

"C'mon, Carroll, honey. You gotta get your beauty sleep if you're going to accept that big old award at Opryland."

They gathered Carroll's belongings and piled into the car. Carroll could not ever remember riding barefoot anywhere but she also could not remember ever before experiencing most of what had happened that evening.

As Peggy's SUV pulled up to the entrance of the Opryland Hotel, Trixie looked over her shoulder into the backseat where Carroll was still wearing her Fan Fair tee-shirt and holding her cashmere sweater set in her hand. The Bally shoes sat beside her on the bench seat. Trixie gave Carroll one more piece of advice. "Honey, don't let the buzzards get you down."

"Trixie, I think it's bastards, not buzzards," sighed Peggy.

"Oh, Lord, honey, whatever. Bastards or buzzards—they're all the same. Now, Dr. Carroll, you put on your shoes and march yourself right into this big old hotel and get yourself in bed. Nothing like a good night's sleep to make a girl feel better. Here, I brought you a couple of my Benadryls to take—course they're Walmart's brand 'cause those ones are cheaper, but you take these and you'll soon be sleeping like a log."

Carroll took the two tiny packages of pink and white capsules and stuck them in her purse, catching a glimpse of the tattered Reconciliation postcard as she made room for the pills in the side pocket.

"Thanks, Trix. And you, too, Peggy. This is a night I won't soon forget."

The three women hugged, and then Peggy and Trixie watched Carroll walk towards the front door of the hotel, pulling her luggage with one hand and holding her sweaters in the other. Peggy began to ease the car gently out of the parking area then braked when she saw Carroll stop and wave just before she walked through the giant front doors of the hotel.

"Wonder if she'll be okay, honey?" Trixie asked.

"I think she'll be fine, Trix," answered Peggy, giving Trixie a pat on the leg, as they drove off.

Carroll closed the door to her hotel room that overlooked the huge indoor conservatory and sat down on the side of the bed, putting her rumpled cashmere twin set beside her on the spread and letting her shoes fall on the floor. She glanced at herself in the mirror over the dresser and shook her head when she saw the transformation wrought earlier in the evening. *This is one for the books*, she thought. The music of a Dixieland band wafted into her room from the atrium below her terrace, and she walked over and closed the veranda doors, her cell phone in hand. The messages light was blinking and she saw that Mitch had called her three times. She punched answer and listened for him to pick up the call.

"You are not going to believe what has happened to me here tonight," she started.

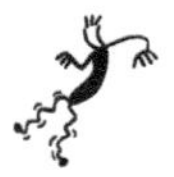

Sunday, May 9, 2004

Chicago

The time at the conference passed quickly, with Carroll greeting the many professional colleagues that stood unanimously in acclaim Sunday morning as she received the award for distinguished work in media representation. As soon as she could do so after the awards luncheon, she headed to the Nashville airport in a hotel van and boarded her flight to Chicago. Enroute the flight attendants presented all mothers on board with their choice of a red or white rose to honor the day. Carroll chose a red one.

She exited the security area in Midway airport, holding her now-wilting rose in her right hand and with her purse slung over her left shoulder, pulling along behind her well-worn black travel suitcase. Hearing a familiar voice calling her name, she strained to look over the heads of her fellow travelers and spotted Janie, waving frantically.

"Hey, Janie. What are you doing here? I thought I told you I would meet you at curbside."

"Hi, Carroll. I'm afraid I have some bad news. You probably don't want to hear it, but I need to tell you that your mother has taken a turn for the worse and isn't expected to live very long. I'll take you to the hospital if you want to go."

Carroll stopped and stood still. Her shoulders sagged and she gulped. Janie eased closer, putting her arm around Carroll's waist.

"I don't know, Janie. It seems so long ago."

"I think you should go, Carroll. There's someone there you need to see. Please let me take you."

"OK. OK. I'm too worn out to resist anymore."

The drive from the airport to the hospital took a short time on this Sunday afternoon, and Carroll and Janie said little to each other during the ride. As they made their way in to the elevator leading to the special care unit, Carroll asked, "What did you mean there's someone there I need to see?"

The doors opened before Janie could respond, and she motioned Carroll to the nearly empty waiting room across the hallway. Although she had not seen her for almost forty years, Carroll immediately recognized Midge, Janie's mother, sitting there next to two other people, a younger woman and a child. As they walked in, Midge stood to greet Carroll with a hug, which Carroll accepted warmly, then Midge blotted her eyes with a cloth handkerchief and squeezed Carroll's hand, before backing away to her seat. The young woman next to Midge looked up and smiled at Carroll.

"Oh my God," Carroll gasped as she looked at the woman and then at the small child sitting next to her. The little girl was drawing pictures in a lined spiral notebook. Her face was turned down, intent on the sketch she was making, and all that was visible to Carroll was a head of curly red ringlets. When the child heard Carroll speak, she looked up, keeping her hand tightly clasped around the pencil in her left hand and the tip of her tongue carefully parked on her upper lip. Her amber eyes squinted in the stark white light of the waiting room as she focused on Carroll.

"Hi," she said. "I'm six-years-old and I'm writing a book about my family. See, here's my mommy and me and my great-grandmother. She's almost dead. I only know how to spell four words, but I can still write a book."

The little girl showed Carroll her carefully written lines of scrolls, each line mimicking cursive handwriting.

Carroll sank into the chair across from the mother and child. Janie stood next to her and said, "Carroll, meet your daughter and granddaughter."

The young woman stood and extended her hand to Carroll. "Hi Carroll—Mom. I'm Michelle—you called me Lisa Ann when I was born. This is my daughter, Caroline," she said, pointing to the youngster.

Carroll looked deeply into the face of the late-thirtyish woman, recognizing the thin lips and aquiline nose and brown eyes, and she knew without a doubt that this was her daughter. The gold crucifix on the chain around the young woman's neck momentarily caught Carroll's eye, then she also stood and reached across the woman's shoulders, gathering her daughter in to her carefully, feeling the resistance of four decades melt away. Both women dissolved into each other for a long moment, then separated slightly looking into each other's faces.

"How? How did you find me?" Carroll finally asked.

Michelle crossed over and they sat down next to each other, holding hands, while Michelle recounted her journey.

"Well, for as long as I can remember, I've known I was adopted. I grew up outside Eugene. My parents had not been able to have children but after they got me they had three biological children, so I was never alone. However, by the time I was in my teens I started wondering who my biological parents had been. Sometimes I would fantasize that I had been left on the doorstep of a church or convent or that my mother had died during childbirth. It was hard for me to get my mind around having been abandoned—given up—but as I got older I realized how many tough choices people have to make as life goes on. Then after I married and had Caroline I wondered where that mop of curly red hair could have come from. Certainly not from me."

Michelle smiled and held up a wisp of her straight brown hair that was clipped short around her oval-shaped face. The two women glanced at the little girl, her serious expression conveying the intensity she seemed to feel as she wrote in her book, her tongue protruding from her mouth on the right side, looking determined to get every word and illustration just right.

Michelle smiled. "She's so serious, so intent. So confident that she can do anything. Don't know where she gets that either—it's certainly not one of my strong suits." She laughed and shifted in the seat.

Hearing the reference to herself, Caroline looked up and said, "My dance recital is next weekend. Would you like to see me do my routine?"

Without waiting for an answer, the little girl stood up, assumed the plié position, and began to perform to the strains of an unheard Music Box Dancer.

The older women applauded and she sat back down and picked up her pencil.

Michelle continued, "You may remember that in the 90's there was a national movement to open up birth records from sealed adoptions. Oregon was one of the first states to do this, and in 2000, I applied for my original birth record to be unsealed. When I received it, I just couldn't stop thinking about what it said. Lisa Ann Murphy—my birth name. My best friend in school had been named Lisa Ann. There was my birth father's name—Robert Barkley. I searched all over Oregon records for someone with that name but nobody came up. Then there was my mother's name—Carol Ann Murphy—C-A-R-O-L—that's how it was spelled. It said you were 17 when you had me, so I decided you must have been in high school, but I could find no records of a Carol Murphy who would have graduated in 1964 in any high school databases in Oregon.

Carroll smiled, and then said softly, "I wasn't from Oregon."

"So I discovered," said Michelle with a grin. "And you didn't really spell your name C-A-R-O-L, either."

Carroll nodded and smiled, dropping her chin and looking up at Michelle with guilt in her eyes.

"The Internet made all the difference. By 2001, I started searching online databases looking for any Carol Ann Murphys who were born in about 1946. Lo and behold one day a ged.com of a Murphy family tree that included a Carroll Ann Murphy—born on October 29, 1946 in Illinois emerged on the search screen. I downloaded it and contacted the woman who had compiled it—that was Frances, your mother.

I told her I was searching for my birth mother and I sent her a photo of Caroline, who was only about three at that time. She immediately sent me back a photo of you at the same age and it was a dead ringer for Caroline. She told me she knew you had gone to Oregon in 1964 but you had severed contact with her then and she knew nothing about your having had a baby, but if it were true, she said, then it would answer a lot of her questions.

I came out to visit her late last year and brought along a photo that I'd seen in the Eugene newspaper a year or so earlier of you receiving the alumni award at OU—it referred to you as Dr. Carroll Ann Murphy, and it had the contents of your acceptance speech and, bingo, we had the rest of the story. We've kept in touch—Frances and I—ever since, and when I learned that her health was deteriorating, I decided to bring Caroline to see her. Mother's Day weekend seemed a fitting time to have our visit. But after I got here on Friday, she became very ill—a heart attack—and has been in the hospital since then. They tell me it doesn't look good for her."

Carroll and Michelle began to cry softly, burrowing their heads in each other's shoulders, while Caroline started to sketch the scene in her notebook. Just then a nurse arrived and announced they should come to Frances' room. "I don't think she has very much longer," the nurse told them, with her eyes downcast. "She's asking for her girls. You can come, too, Caroline."

Midge and Janie stayed behind in the waiting room, grabbing tattered magazines through which they slowly began flipping pages.

Michelle held Caroline's left hand while Carroll held the right one, and they walked down the short corridor towards Frances' hospital room. Carroll noticed the prominent Do Not Resuscitate sign posted at the entrance and smiled to herself. *That's Frances—the nurse to the end.*

Frances' head lay on the pillow with an oxygen cannula resting in her nostrils. Her face was very pale and her breaths were shallow and uneven. An IV dripped slowly into a vein in her left arm and a heart monitor showed a slow but regular cadence. As the small family group entered, Frances opened her eyes a little, trying to take in the vision of the three succeeding generations of women who stood there.

"Carroll," she mouthed hoarsely.

The nurse handed Carroll a small cup filled with thickened liquid and urged Carroll to offer it to her mother. As Carroll placed the cup next to her mother's lips, Frances took a little of the fluid on the tip of her tongue and licked her dry lips.

"Hello, Mother." Carroll smiled and patted her mother's shrunken hand. The coolness of it startled Carroll, who momentarily let it go, and then re-grasped it.

"I wish I'd known," Frances said, able to speak a little more audibly now.

"I wish I could have told you. I'm sorry." She patted her mother's hand and received a small squeeze in return.

"Me, too. At least I held on long enough to see you all together one time," Frances said, smiling slightly as she urged the words out of her worn-out throat. "Now I can die at peace. Love you."

Frances shut her eyes and her breathing paused.

"Love you, too."

Carroll continued to hold her mother's cool hand waiting for her to take another breath, and then the monitor alarm sounded as Frances heartbeat slowed to almost nothing, and then became a flat line. Carroll, Michelle, and Caroline held each other's hands and wept as their ancestor transitioned. The nurse shut off the alarm and stepped out of the room.

Caroline spoke first, "I think she's gone to heaven, Mommy."

"Yes, I think so, too, Carrie honey. Let's pray for her."

As Midge and Janie entered the room accompanied by the nurse, they were astonished to see two curly red-heads and one brown one, bowed down, while they recited in unison "Our father who art in heaven...."

The five of them left the hospital together to walk to Janie's car, Caroline holding her mother's hand. As they neared the parking lot the little girl looked up at her mother and asked, "Is it still Mother's Day, Mommy, even though Granny Fran is dead?"

"Yes, honey, it's still Mother's Day," her mother answered.

"Are you my real mommy?"

"Yes, honey, I am."

"And were you inside Carroll's tummy before you were born?"

“Yes, on that, too, sweetie. She’s my birth mommy and Grandma Ellen back in Oregon is the mommy who raised me.”

“I love having another grandma, Mommy.”

Caroline began to skip and dance ahead of the women, finding her way to Janie’s car before anyone else. As they waited for Janie to unlock the car doors, Carroll bent down and picked up the little girl, holding her tight. Caroline snuggled her nose into Carroll’s fuzzy hair, and Carroll said, “Dearest Caroline, this is the best gift any mother or grandmother could ever receive on Mother’s Day.”

She reached out to hug Michelle, enfolding Caroline between them. Unentangling herself, Michelle reached in to the back seat of Janie’s car.

“I have something else for you, Mom,” she said. “When I was with Frances Friday before she got so sick, she gave me these and asked me to give them to you if I ever met you. I think they are her journals.”

“Oh my God,” said Carroll for the second time today.

She lifted the lid on the cardboard box and removed the top notebook, which displayed the notice, For Carroll’s Eyes Only. Flipping to the last entry, she saw Frances still familiar though shakily scrawled cursive handwriting.

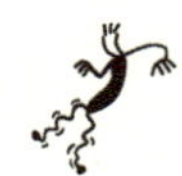

May 7, 2004

Dearest Carroll

I can hardly believe I am a great-grandmother. Great-grandmother! And I didn't even know I was a grandmother until a few months ago. Our grandchildren redeem us, I think, because we can get it right with them where we may have failed with our children.

How sad for you and me that the birth of your daughter came between us all these years. I have longed for you for forty years, and I can't help but believe you have longed for your lost daughter all this time, too.

And now Michelle and Caroline are coming to see me. If only you could be here, too.

You are my precious beloved daughter.

Love always,

Mother

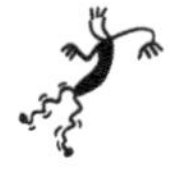

The End

Acknowledgements

This book has been in the works for twelve years. The airplane scene with the Trollops, which was the first of many, came to me in 2004 as I sat in the nursing home beside the bed of my dying mother. During that dark period, I wrote in my journal on a regular basis to distract me from the conflicting emotions I was feeling as I watched her move several times towards and then away from her transition from earth, an event she had said for several years she was looking forward to doing. Although I didn't recognize it for what it was at the time, I'm quite sure now she couldn't die until I got right with her dying, and in order for me to do that, I had to work through a number of mother-daughter issues about which we had conflicted over time. Since she was not available to participate in these resolutions, I think Trixie, Peggy, and Carroll came along to help me out. I wrote the forty pages of their airplane ride during those weeks.

A few months later I saw a notice in the local newspaper about an upcoming workshop for prospective writers and I enrolled. When I showed up for the class and was asked in what genre I wrote, I couldn't answer that question because I didn't know what a genre was.

The workshop was led by members of the Council for the Written Word of Williamson County. I took in every morsel they offered and signed on immediately to their weekly writer's critique group. Sally R. Lee and Louise Coln who facilitated that group endured every word of the girls' plane travel, read aloud, during those early months. For years afterward they would ask if everybody finally got off that plane. Thanks, ladies, and to all the other members of the CWW who read or heard innumerable versions of the story and offered great suggestions.

Among the writers I met at that first writing workshop in 2004 I was most impressed by two ladies. River Jordan was selling *The Gin Girl*, her first novel. I was awed to speak to a published author and I confided my hopes for my novel. She responded so warmly and with so much encouragement and I have never forgotten her generosity. Currie Alexander Powers was fairly new to the writing community in 2004 but she had great skills. She soon published *Soul of a Man* which is one of my top ten favorite books. In 2009 she edited my first book, *Gotcha Covered: A Legacy of Service and Protection.* I am so grateful for the terrific blurb Currie gave me for *Proud Flesh.*

The title of the book comes from a southern colloquialism used to describe a medical condition in humans when a wound does not properly heal, causing it to weep. I first heard the term in the 1970's from a patient in reference to a tumor protruding through her skin and subsequently heard it used by other patients to describe non-healing conditions. It seemed an apt phrase for the various life maladies these girls experienced.

In the fall of 2006 I decided the book was finished and I began seeking agent representation. Twenty letters went out to prestigious agents and twenty rejections quickly followed. Then Louise suggested I might try a local agent, newly in business but not new to books. Angela DePriest called me the day she received my inquiry and wanted to know where I had been hiding. She said she hadn't stopped laughing since the manuscript arrived. We signed soon after and at her suggestion the book went into editorial review with Jamie Chavez, who was incredibly talented. Efforts by DePriest to sell the book to publishing houses came to a screeching halt with the arrival of the recession of 2008 and sadly our relationship ended, but I will always be grateful that she saw something in me to encourage me to keep plodding along. I'm also grateful to Chavez, whose sound edits were always accompanied by the caveat, "Remember we are on the same team."

Version after version followed, and then one day nothing further would come. I took the problem to critique group and someone suggested maybe I was trying too hard to tell a story and not hard enough to hear my characters tell me their story. That afternoon I called all the girls together in a group and asked if this were true. It was, and they were not willing to tell me more if I were determined to have the story end my way and not their way. Trixie thought I was looking down on her and especially on her little, bitty, baby dog, and she was having none of it. I apologized and agreed to channel their story and not try to control it, though they conceded I could add grammar and could occasionally shorten some particularly long tale. And so we wrote on and the end came out fairly quickly. It seems since Carroll had never told her story to anyone, she had lots of fear in being outed, but it all ended well.

In about 2009 while vacationing in Mexico I spoke with a fellow vacationer, Kathy Biagi, who knew someone who had graduated from Oregon in Carroll's class. Tresa Eyres, a writer and radio journalist in San Francisco, read the Duck part and shared with me her class yearbooks from the period which helped me fill in the background on Eugene and the campus scene in the late 1960's. She corrected my timeline and added a little personal color and I am very grateful. Dianne Gannaway Greene patiently copy edited an early version and told me she loved the book, which meant a lot from someone who reads books regularly in her professional capacity.

On several occasions I tried to find another agent who could represent my writing to a big publisher. One of the hoped-for-agents, someone in New York, told me there was no way people such as my characters actually existed. I knew she'd never been to a WalMart in the south on a Saturday. Another said this reads like non-fiction turned into fiction. I think hardly any fiction writers make it all up. All of us are constantly eavesdropping on life, whether we are riding a plane, a bus, or a streetcar; whether attending a funeral, a wedding, or a graduation. Occasionally, in a life-imitates-art kind of sense, something falls into our lap and the event is too good to not stow away just waiting for the right story to fit it into. The last airplane scene with "Ronnie" happened exactly as I wrote it. Thanks to all the other folks from whom I might have borrowed a smidgeon.

Along the way more people read the story and reacted to it. Some loved Trixie, some loved Peggy, but only a few loved Carroll. "She's not a very sympathetic protagonist," one said. How can a reader root for a main character that is so darn hardened on the outside and only in a tiny way allows a reader to see her vulnerable inside? Melody Lawrence, a literary critic in New York, who very much believed in the girls, read the manuscript and suggested I find some way to connect Carroll's seemingly cool persona with the always warm one of Trixie. I had a hard time getting Carroll to show some softness, but then I realized it was in the tiniest ways she showed her compassionate character--through clipping Barbara's flowers, for instance. If you have arrived this far in the book, you probably found enough about her to at least like her a little before her final meltdown. Thanks for hanging in there with her.

At a Christmas party in Nashville in 2014, Alice Randall asked me what I was writing and I told her I had just finished what I hoped would be the final draft to my first novel. She asked me to send it to her so she could write a blurb. I barely got home from the party before I zipped it off to her and she graciously sent the blurb soon after the first of the year. Thanks, Alice.

There actually *are* three charter Trollops whose beginning came about at a family wedding when we were all outed. I'll own being T#1 but T#2 and T#3 will need to claim their own places for themselves. Numbers 4-11 are very out and about in the Alpha chapter, however, having been initiated as official T's. They have even purchased their very own Keds and white ankle socks. Thanks, Sara, Julie, Marilyn, Suzanne, Linda, Elaine, Sally, and Mary Catharine, and to Marti, from afar--for your love and support. It's easy being easy with you girls.

Along the way of this writing journey I learned that more than 99% of readers choose a novel by its cover. As I moved toward publication I worked with several people of the BFF variety who helped shape my thinking about this cover. At a writing critique group meeting in Franklin in the fall of 2015, I saw a cover of a recently published book from Westview designed partially by the artist and writer, Sandy Zeigler. Impressed by the way it looked like a "real book" I sought Sandy's input on my upcoming cover. She offered wonderful suggestions that moved me along the line to finding a professional graphics designer specializing in cover designs. Tim Park, a childhood friend and fellow Maryville High School class of 1962 graduate, whose career in graphic design has taken him to great heights, offered to give this a shot despite having never designed a book cover. At the same time, he strongly urged me to go with someone whose career specializes in designing these covers. That direction led me to Eddie Patton, whose terrific cover design you are holding in your hands. Thanks to all my guides along the way who helped keep me from stumbling down my own path.

We know there are many, many other T's and T wannabes out there. We even know some have died while the book was being written else they would be dancing in their white Keds today. We miss them and honor them, and we welcome new chapters and members. You can make up your own rituals and initiations, but do try to wear your white Keds and try to do a little dancing--it's therapy for your broken heart.

In the late 1990's when I was just past the fifty year mark someone gave me a copy of the hottest new novel then on the Best Seller list. I read the book with great difficulty because I found it so uninteresting and so predictable, but mostly I found it to be without the wisdom that comes from living past age fifty. I hope you will tell about a hundred of your friends and their friends that this is a book to which almost all women who came of age in the 1960's and 1970's can relate. This could be any of our stories.

Ginger Manley
Franklin, Tennessee
April 2016

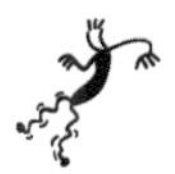

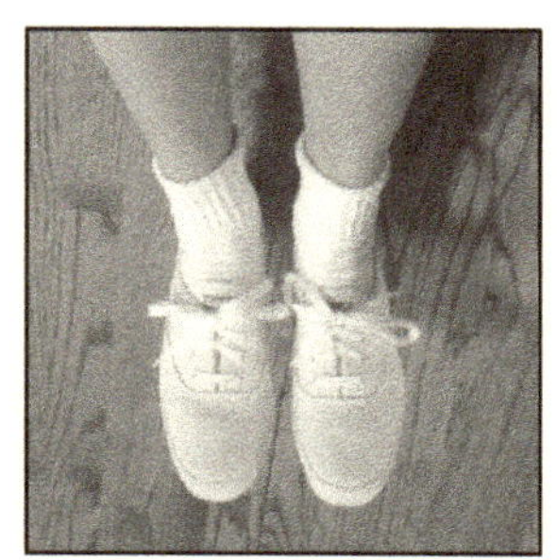

About the Author

Ginger Manley grew up in Appalachia and writes today from her home outside Nashville, TN. She is still trying to answer the question about what genre she writes in, but having completed four books in four different categories, she is pretty sure she will never know the answer. *Proud Flesh* is a novel--of that she's certain. The others are an anthology, a self-help book, and a memoir.

When she is not confused about genre, she teaches doctors and nurses from all over the country how to behave appropriately in the work place. She has had an active career as a nurse practitioner and sex therapist for almost fifty years and she feels honored to have been a part of so many journeys in that capacity.

In her spare time, she enjoys travel with her husband of more than forty-eight years and the occasional reunion with the Trollops. She is still trying to learn to breathe while swinging a golf club and even though she has had both of her knee joints replaced she will still start to flat-foot at the first note of *Rocky Top* or of any other piece of old-time mountain music.

She can be reached at ginger@gingermanley.com.

Trixie blogs at www.proudfleshbook.com.